# What Happened in the Woodshed

# What Happened in the Woodshed

## The Secret Lives of Battered Children and a New Profession to Protect Them

Lawrence R. Ricci, MD

*Foreword by Stephen Ludwig, MD*

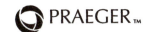 PRAEGER™

An Imprint of ABC-CLIO, LLC

Santa Barbara, California • Denver, Colorado

**Library of Congress Cataloging-in-Publication Data**

Names: Ricci, Lawrence R., author.
Title: What happened in the woodshed : the secret lives of battered children
    and a new profession to protect them / Lawrence R. Ricci, MD ; foreword
    by Stephen Ludwig, MD.
Description: Santa Barbara, California : Praeger, [2018] | Includes bibliographical
    references and index.
Identifiers: LCCN 2017056367 (print) | LCCN 2017058507 (ebook) |
    ISBN 9781440856372 (ebook) | ISBN 9781440856365 (alk. paper)
Subjects: LCSH: Child abuse—United States. | Abused children—United States. |
    Abused children—Health risk assessment—United States. | Pediatrics—
    United States. | Child welfare—United States.
Classification: LCC HV6626.52 (ebook) | LCC HV6626.52 .R524 2018 (print) |
    DDC 362.760973—dc23
LC record available at https://lccn.loc.gov/2017056367

ISBN: 978-1-4408-5636-5 (print)
      978-1-4408-5637-2 (ebook)

22 21 20 19 18    1 2 3 4 5

This book is also available as an eBook.

Praeger
An Imprint of ABC-CLIO, LLC

ABC-CLIO, LLC
130 Cremona Drive, P.O. Box 1911
Santa Barbara, California 93116-1911
www.abc-clio.com

This book is printed on acid-free paper ∞

Manufactured in the United States of America

*For my parents Ron and Mae Ricci who kept me safe
in an unsafe world.*

*For my wife Laurel Ricci who showed me that sometimes
the world can be safe.*

A solemn consideration, when I enter a great city by night, that every one of those darkly clustered houses encloses its own secret; that every room in every one of them encloses its own secret; that every beating heart in the hundreds of thousands of breasts, there is, in some of its imaginings, a secret to the heart nearest it!

—Charles Dickens, *A Tale of Two Cities*, 1859

# Contents

*Foreword by Stephen Ludwig, MD*  xi

*Acknowledgments*  xiii

*Prologue: Danny: What Happened in the Woodshed?*  xv

*Introduction: The Secret Lives of Battered Children*  xvii

**Chapter 1**  The Making of a Child Abuse Pediatrician
and the Birth of a New Specialty  1

**Chapter 2**  Mistakes: It Could Be Anyone  19

**Chapter 3**  Down the Rabbit Hole with Baron Munchausen  33

**Chapter 4**  The Hidden Ravages of Neglect  47

**Chapter 5**  Child Abuse Fatalities: The Anatomy of Death  63

**Chapter 6**  Failure to Protect: The Taking of Justice  79

**Chapter 7**  A Parent's Grief: Pam and Benji  93

**Chapter 8**  The Courtroom: Triumph of Style over Substance  105

**Chapter 9**  Vicarious Trauma: "How Can You Do This Work?"  121

**Chapter 10**  The Future of Our Children: Child Abuse
Prevention in America and Internationally  137

*Epilogue: Strider: What Happened in the Woodshed!*  149

*Appendix: Child Abuse Doctors Who Shared Their Stories*          153

*References*                                                                              159

*Index*                                                                                       165

# Foreword

This book unveils the harsh reality of hidden abuses that children encounter and also takes us along on the mission of a new breed of amazing men and women who have dedicated their careers to detecting and protecting these most vulnerable members of our society.

As a third year medical student in 1969, I walked into a Grand Rounds Conference at St. Christopher's Hospital for Children being given by a pediatrician named Dr. Ray Helfer. That talk would change my life. It was a presentation about child abuse, which was, at the time, not widely recognized by either medicine or the wider public. I was captivated. I wanted to know more, but information on the topic was scarce.

Years later, I was a pediatric resident at the Children's Hospital National Medical Center in Washington, DC. There, child abuse became reality to me in the emergency room, clinic, and inpatient service. It was no longer theoretical. It was real, sometimes even a life and death issue. Working with fellow residents, social workers, nurses, and faculty, we started a child abuse team in 1971 to better care for the scores of abused and neglected children we saw each year. Later, at the Children's Hospital of Philadelphia, I continued my care of abused children, on an intense quest to learn more about the how and why of this abuse and neglect, and what could help protect these children.

As time passed, I learned a great deal about abuse. I worked with almost every specialty and subspecialty group of physicians, nurses, social workers, community workers, child protective service workers, police, lawyers, judges, and parents. What was once the mystery of child abuse became clearer, although no less sad. I helped train some younger colleagues who have now become career specialists in the care of abused and neglected children, some of whom have gone on to especially distinguished careers and are contributors to this book. During those years, throughout the United States and the world, like-minded professional also took up the mission. As their numbers increased, we formed the Helfer Society, named after that man who was my first "teacher" on the problem of child abuse and also my inspiration to take action against it. We ultimately, in 2009, created a distinct pediatric subspecialty—child abuse pediatrics.

This book's editor, Larry Ricci, MD, was at the forefront of that movement. He too had seen the results of abuse and was determined to make a difference. This volume is just one manifestation of his career devoted to children and families.

*What Happened in the Woodshed* tells the stories of children who have been abused, and the stories of their families. Their usually secret lives shared here show the range of the effects of abuse, from the physical and sexual to neglect, or Munchausen, and to the fatal. The second vital narrative in this text is that of the professional response, the stories of those men and women on a mission, and the scientific work that has been done to advance our understanding of abuse and neglect, hopefully leading closer to prevention and amelioration of pain, disability, and death.

Still, even today, there remain some "abuse nay-sayers." These are people who do not believe that abuse occurs, or who think that there are other explanations for the scientifically proven evidence of abuse. They are often "legal experts" who do not have medical or research expertise. The child abuse professionals and their work chronicled in this text are not here to judge these individuals. That judgment will come in time.

First and last, this book is the story of its editor, Dr. Ricci, who is a combination of great passion and compassion. His honesty and commitment fill every page. I thank Dr. Ricci for such a wonderful contribution. This volume is a tribute to his work.

Yes, things do happen in the woodshed, the home, the apartment, and elsewhere. This book is a must read for all medical students, physicians, nurses, health care, and law enforcement professionals. And it is a must read for informed citizens, neighbors, and relatives.

Stephen Ludwig, MD
Professor of Pediatrics
Perelman School of Medicine
University of Pennsylvania
Philadelphia, PA
2017

# Acknowledgments

Just as child abuse work requires a multidisciplinary team, writing this book required a multidisciplinary team. First and foremost, I must thank Debbie Carvalko, my editor at Praeger. I spoke with many editors and agents about this book over the last few years. Almost without exception, I was told that no one would want to read a book about child abuse. Debbie was the exception.

After I submitted my proposal to her, she quickly wrote back that Praeger wanted to publish the book, not as a child abuse pediatrician's memoir as I had originally envisioned it, but as a compendium of the voices of many child abuse pediatricians. Her vision opened an intriguing door for me to explore the personal and professional stories of many of my colleagues, stories that would otherwise never have been told. Debbie has, as any good editor, challenged and supported me along the way. Her advice has made this book so much better than it would have been otherwise.

I must thank the 30 child abuse pediatricians listed in the appendix who allowed me to interview them. They generously gave their time and their hearts. I hope the reader appreciates their stories as much as I have. In particular, I have to thank Dr. Robert Reece who not only encouraged me in the writing of this book but who has been a steadfast mentor throughout my career. Dr. David Kerns also helped me with his sage advice. I am also appreciative of the assistance the library staff at Maine Medical Center provided me in my almost daily request for articles, some obscure and hard to find. I must also express my appreciation for Doctor David Chadwick's series of child abuse doctor biographies in his book, *The Child Abuse Doctors* published by STM Learning.

This book is about pediatricians who specialize in the care of abused children. But pediatricians are not the only ones who help abused children. Other professions help these children as well. Child protective workers, law enforcement professionals, other medical and mental health professionals have stories that are equally important and that should be told.

In particular, I must thank Pam Belisle and Benji Wilber for allowing me to listen to and retell their stories of losing a child at the hands of another. These touching stories of loss, even now so many years later, were difficult for them to share, and difficult for me to listen to. Thank you Pam and Benji.

This book has been several years in the making. Over those years, I received invaluable help from a number of writing professionals, colleagues, friends, and at least three family members.

Early on, Rita Robinson from Writer's Digest University helped me learn to keep on topic and on deadline. Later, I attended a writing seminar for medical providers at Harvard titled "Writing, Publishing, and Social Media for Health Care Professionals." It was here that I met Debbie Carvalko. It was here that I also met Margaret Murphy who helped me with my book proposal. Joseph Stinson, a former high school friend and now a Hollywood screenwriter, also gave me invaluable support and assistance with the proposal.

Though not particularly germane to the book itself, I could not have done the child abuse pediatrics work, which ultimately led to this book, without the help of so many colleagues over the past 30 years. I have to single out Bruce Cummings, former maternal and child health administrator at Mid-Maine Medical Center in Waterville, Maine; Dick Watson, social worker at Maine General Medical Center in Augusta, Maine; Sandi Hodge, former director of Maine Child Welfare; and David Crook, former district attorney of Maine's Kennebec and Somerset Counties. Harvey Berman and Jack Rosser, former directors at Spurwink, supported me in my program and career development when I moved from Waterville to Portland, Maine. I also must thank my many current colleagues, in particular, Joyce Wientzen, program director for the Spurwink Child Abuse Program, and Eric Meyer, executive director at Spurwink.

Finally, I must thank my daughter Ariel Ricci who honed her editorial skills in London and who has reviewed and edited this book several times, my sister-in-law Lynn Webber who first suggested the cover idea of a woodshed, and my wife Laurel Ricci for not only reading the book but for thinking of me as a good writer. Writing is not easy, especially for those of us unskilled at it. While I have struggled to learn its intricacies, a supportive voice can buoy me for days, weeks, months, even years. Thank you, my beautiful family.

# Prologue: Danny: What Happened in the Woodshed?

In 1984, just as I was beginning my career as a child abuse pediatrician, I spoke at a public library about the medical diagnosis of child abuse. The audience was small, maybe 15 people, surrounded by row after row of children's books. Some in the audience were child welfare professionals, some were nonprofessional community members. All were there, I hoped, to learn about child abuse and, in particular, about my new program— the Pediatric Forensic Clinic. I described how that program would help protect children by providing an accurate medical diagnosis, sometimes finding that a child had been abused and making sure the child was protected, sometimes finding that a child had not been abused and saving the family from further investigation.

Afterward, as I prepared to leave, a well-dressed, elderly woman approached me. Tall and thin, with grey hair and a sad, wrinkled face, she stood rigidly, her eyes fixed on the floor. In a halting whisper, she told me a story I would never forget.

When her son Danny was a toddler and misbehaved, as toddlers often do, her now deceased husband would roughly haul him into the wood-shed. This happened often, sometimes daily. After a time, Danny and his father would come back. But on returning, her usually noisy, rambunctious son would be quiet and withdrawn. He would sometimes whimper, sometimes cower. He would, more often than not, curl into his mother's lap and quietly fall asleep. Sometimes, he slept for an interminably long time and, even after he awoke, he seemed groggy, almost punch-drunk. Sometimes, his mother saw bruises on his face. Sometimes, when she dared to look, she saw bruises on his buttocks.

She would try to nurse her damaged son back to health by holding and rocking him. What else was she to do? In the 1950s, there was no one for her to turn to for help. There were no child welfare agencies, no public education campaigns, no protective physicians or teachers. Even had there been, Danny never left his home.

I tried then but could not picture that woodshed or what happened in it. But now, after 30 years of seeing literally thousands of abused children, I think I might know what happened to Danny, if only because of what I have since learned from other children's experiences, including those literally taken into the woodshed.

I can see it now, like so many other woodsheds—dark, except when lit by a propane lantern casting harsh shadows on the bare, unfinished walls, cold, except when warmed by a woodstove, dingy with dirt floor and rusty, seldom used tools amidst overflowing ashtrays, and empty beer cans. The atmosphere would have been oppressive, even horrifying, for a two-year-old boy who knew what was coming next.

Danny's mother never asked her husband what happened in that woodshed. She never spoke about it to him or anyone else. Gradually, over the ensuing years, a terrible realization came over her. Danny, now an adult, is profoundly mentally handicapped. She told me, as her eyes filled and her voice broke, that after hearing me speak about abusive head trauma and its effect on a baby's brain, she was now certain that her son's brain had been damaged by what was done to him in that woodshed.

I have often thought about that mother and her story. I have wondered, as she did, what happened to Danny in that woodshed. No one will ever know. Danny can't speak and his father is dead. His mother saw the aftermath but could not begin to imagine the worst of it.

# Introduction:
# The Secret Lives of Battered Children

Child abuse is the greatest secret of all. It is a secret to family members who don't see it, to professionals who don't understand it, to politicians who neither see nor understand it. But child abuse is not a secret to everyone. *What Happened in the Woodshed* is a detective story of how well-trained and experienced child abuse pediatricians can deduce, much like Sherlock Holmes, how an injury was inflicted from the injury itself. The crime scene of a child's abused and neglected body can, through careful medical analysis, lead us inexorably back to what happened, sometimes to who did it, and most revealingly to why it happened.

Told through the eyes of child abuse pediatricians, *What Happened in the Woodshed* is a book about some of the abused and neglected children I and my colleagues have seen, not all of them of course, but the most compelling of so many compelling cases. Some cases will always feel fresh in our minds even after many years, not only because of their severity but because of their lasting impact on us personally and professionally. Perhaps disproportionately, we talk about dead babies, battered babies, starved and neglected babies. This is not intended to shock, though shocking these cases may be, nor is it intended to ignore the many children who are abused in other ways. But, rather our intent is to describe our own most compelling experiences.

Among my own cases, there is the 14-year-old boy lying on his death bed. His mother buys a cemetery plot, family gathers around, but something isn't quite right. How was it that his sibling had died years earlier from a similar mysterious illness, one that even then raised questions about intentional poisoning?

A seven-year-old boy comes into the hospital weighing 20 pounds, having not seen a doctor nor not gained any weight in several years. How and why did this happen?

A four-month-old boy comes into the hospital to die from abuse. How was it that during his few months of life, more than 15 professionals in five agencies failed to protect him?

A mother receives the most dreaded call of all. Her infant son had stopped breathing at the babysitter's home. He later dies from abusive head trauma. What can this mother's unspeakable grief tell us about devastating sorrow and ultimate empowerment?

All of my and my colleagues' stories are true. I have tried diligently and I hope successfully to mask identifying details, while striving to preserve essential facts and concepts. Some stories, though, are drawn from public news and court records. This is true of Ricky, Logan, and Strider.

These stories are not academic. They are, rather, deeply personal. It is this very personal view that I hope will project the reality of child abuse from our eyes to the readers. It is this view that hopefully will reveal not just what happened to these children but what these children and families can teach us about all children before they become damaged and sometimes damaging adults.

This book is not intended to be a systematic review of either the history or the science of child abuse. Nor is it intended as a critique of any system or individual. We all make mistakes. However, I honestly believe that everyone, parents and professionals alike, do their best with what they have.

*What Happened in the Woodshed* is a book about good parents and bad, about good outcomes and bad, about perpetrators and victims, and, not least, about collateral victims, the family members who did not cause the abuse and the professionals who identify and treat the abuse.

*What Happened in the Woodshed* is not just my story and that of my child abuse pediatrician colleagues, it is also the story of the emergence and development of child abuse pediatrics as a formal pediatric specialty in 2006.

Ultimately though, *What Happened in the Woodshed* is for and about Danny. It is my attempt to bear witness to Danny's story by way of other stories of abused children, to try to fathom who these children are, who their parents are, and, with as much precision as is medically possible, tell what happened to them in the many secret and silent homes in America where children are abused and neglected every day.

## CHAPTER ONE

# The Making of a Child Abuse Pediatrician and the Birth of a New Specialty

Child abuse pediatrics did not begin in 2006 when the American Board of Pediatrics formally recognized it as a certified specialty of pediatrics. Its origins can be traced back to the late 19th century with the published work of one physician, French forensic pathologist Ambroise Tardieu. Prior to his publications, child abuse as a medical phenomenon, or even as a social one, was rarely described, much less recognized, and there were vanishingly few references to child abuse in the medical literature of the past two centuries (Lynch 1985). Most injuries to infants and children were presumed to be accidents, sometimes self-inflicted, or occasionally inflicted by other children, but never inflicted by an adult caretaker. The terms "child abuse" and "battered child syndrome" had not yet come into existence.

Ambroise Tardieu was a professor of forensic medicine at the University of Paris who published three detailed studies on child abuse. Yet, even with these remarkable studies, child abuse would be ignored by medical science for another 100 years until the publication of papers in the United States in the mid-20th century.

Tardieu's work itself was only formally recognized with the presentation on September 20, 2003, of "Ambroise Tardieu: The Man and His Work on Child Maltreatment a Century Before Kempe" by Doctor Jean Labbe, a pediatrician from Laval University Quebec, Canada, to the Ray Helfer Society, an international society of child abuse physicians.

Labbe's presentation was followed in 2005 by two papers in the journal *Child Abuse & Neglect* (Labbe 2005; Roche et al. 2005). *Child Abuse & Neglect: The International Journal* was started in 1977 by the International Society for the Prevention of Child Abuse and Neglect. It was the first peer-reviewed journal to focus exclusively on child abuse.

In *Forensic Study on Offenses against Morals* published in 1857, Tardieu described almost 1,000 cases of sexual abuse, mostly in children (Tardieu 1857; Labbe 2005). This paper was far ahead of its time for its lucid description of injuries caused by sexual abuse. It also contained drawings of normal and abnormal genital findings, presaging the photo documentation and anatomic descriptions of such injuries in the United States in the 1980s. Tardieu noted that, even if abuse was proven to have occurred such as by confession, the physical examination could be normal if enough time had passed for healing to occur. Even now, many child abuse pediatricians are asked in court and elsewhere why an examination might be normal in a child who had been sexually abused. Tardieu believed abuse most likely was perpetrated by a parent in the very home where the child lived. Everything that Tardieu described in 1857 about sexual abuse would lie hidden for more than a century, eventually rediscovered by child abuse pediatricians in the United States in the early 1980s.

In 1860, Tardieu published "Forensic Study on Cruelty and the Ill-Treatment of Children" (Tardieu 1860; Labbe 2005). The paper described 32 battered children, 18 of whom died. This work foreshadowed the seminal paper "The Battered Child Syndrome" published by Henry Kempe and colleagues 100 years later (Kempe et al. 1962).

Finally, Tardieu authored a book in 1868, *Forensic Study on Infanticide* (Tardieu 1868; Labbe 2005), based on the study of over 500 infants, mostly newborns, all of whom were suffocated by their mothers.

In the introduction to his 1860 paper, Tardieu reported, "Among the many and diverse cases of which is composed the topic of medico-legal [having to do with the intersection of medicine and the law] injuries, there is a group altogether different from the rest, and which, hidden in obscurity until the present day, deserves a thorough unveiling. I wish to speak of those deeds, described as acts of cruelty and ill treatment, of which young children fall victim from their parents, their schoolmasters, and all of who exert over these children some degree of authority" (Roche et al. 2005, 326).

Later he added, "From the earliest days of their lives, such piteous defenseless beings are destined each day, each hour even, for the cruelest of abuse, are submitted to harsh deprivations, their lives hardly begun are already a martyrdom, such torment, such physical tortures from which the imagination recoils lay waste their bodies, extinguishes the first awakenings of their minds and cuts short their very lives" (Roche et al. 2005, 326). Many child abuse doctors I spoke to for this book even now speak of that same horror.

Tardieu noted that most of the cases he reported involved very young children under the age of 3. He described how wasted and sad these children were, "dazed with vacant gaze." Once these children were protected and nurtured, their improvement in appearance and demeanor astounded him.

Presaging the modern analysis of inflicted injuries in children, Tardieu described bruises of varying color suggesting multiple assault, bruises with hand and weapon imprints, and bruises over parts of the body not normally injured in play, such as the face and back. Remarkably, he even described subdural hematomas (blood clots on the surface of the brain from trauma) of dead children. This later finding would not be revisited until the 1950s with the work of John Caffey.

Tardieu warned physicians against "incorrect conclusions from the examination of such individuals and against the habitual explanations proffered by those who are the authors of these grave lesions." He denounced the claim by perpetrators of the right to parental discipline, if only because of the disproportion between the misdeed and the punishment.

Tardieu hoped that his work would be the basis for a revolution in the care and protection of abused children. What then was the scientific and public impact of these landmark papers? There was none. Unfortunately, his work was completely ignored, perhaps because society, at that time, considered family affairs private and children property, perhaps because there had always been the belief among adults that children are habitual liars.

Not only was Tardieu's work ignored and soon forgotten but for the next century little was written about abusive injuries. Then in 1946, John Caffey, an American pediatric radiologist, published a paper describing several children with multiple fractures and subdural hematomas (Caffey 1946). Although it is said he suspected abuse, Caffey did not report this in his paper, rather he offered that the cause was unknown but likely traumatic. He reported that the trauma was denied by the caretaker and that such denial was of unclear motivation, as if parents were, for unknown reason, unwilling or unable to describe a serious, presumably accidental injury.

Frederic Silverman, also a pediatric radiologist, published "The Roentgen Manifestations of Unrecognized Skeletal Trauma in Infants" (Silverman 1953). He described three children with multiple old and new fractures he believed were secondary to unrecognized trauma. Like Caffey before him, he would not go so far as to diagnose abuse. However, in a 1994 invited letter to the editor of the journal *Pediatric Radiology*, Silverman stated that both he and Caffey, at the time of their publications, strongly suspected that the cause of these injuries was abuse but did not say that because of fear of legal repercussions (Silverman 1994). Only later, after Henry Kempe and colleagues put the name "battered child syndrome" to what was happening to these children, were the floodgates opened and what was obscure in the publications of Caffey, Silverman, and others finally revealed for what it truly was, child abuse.

In 1962, Henry Kempe, a pediatrician at Denver Children's Hospital, along with his colleagues, published the seminal paper "The Battered Child Syndrome" and everything changed (Kempe et al. 1962). After that publication, national news outlets began covering the story.

Kempe was quoted in *Newsweek* saying, "One day last November we had four battered children in our pediatrics ward. Two died in the hospital and one died four weeks later at home. For every child who enters the hospital this badly beaten, there must be hundreds treated by unsuspecting doctors. The battered child syndrome isn't a reportable disease, but it damn well ought to be" (*Newsweek* 1962, 74).

Kempe and his colleagues were in the forefront of the development of the modern child welfare system and the mandatory reporting law, now in all 50 states. They identified 749 abuse victims in their survey of hospitals and district attorney offices. In the most recent National Incidence Study, more than 1.25 million children in the United States are abused each year, while an additional 1.75 million are at significant risk of abuse.

Child sexual abuse was not formally recognized as a medical problem until 1977, when Kempe published "Sexual Abuse, Another Hidden Pediatric Problem" (Kempe 1978). At the same time, researchers and advocates became interested in violence against women and, by extension, violence against children. Across the nation, women were being asked about childhood abuse. Astonishingly, one in five said they had been sexually abused as children. These researchers and therapists then turned to children and asked them the same question. The same unimaginable percentage of children reported that they had indeed been sexually abused, usually in their own home, just as Tardieu had said.

These children, once identified, not only needed mental health treatment, but they needed a skilled medical examination to look for signs of trauma and infection. It was this incredible volume of newly identified sexually abused children pouring into emergency rooms and pediatric offices around the country that directly led to the beginning of the new field of child abuse pediatrics. Because they took an interest in the care

of these children, a number of physicians, mostly pediatricians, were recruited to examine them. Child welfare workers would send children to these physicians who took it on themselves to develop together expertise in this new area of medicine.

In 1996, Steven Ludwig, professor of pediatrics at Children's Hospital of Philadelphia, convened a group of pediatricians including myself, Bob Reece (professor of pediatrics, TUFTS University Boston), Howard Dubowitz (professor of pediatrics, University of Maryland), Cindy Christian (professor of pediatrics, Children's Hospital of Philadelphia), and Des Runyon (professor of pediatrics, University of North Carolina) to talk about developing a specialty. In 1997, the first national meeting of child abuse pediatricians was held in Philadelphia (Ricci et al. 2002). In 2006, the American Board of Pediatrics approved the new specialty of child abuse pediatrics. In 2010, 191 pediatricians, who took and passed the board-certifying examination, were recognized as child abuse pediatricians. As of 2017, there are close to 400 board-certified child abuse pediatricians in the United States, a good start but not nearly enough.

---

Like Tardieu, Caffey, Silverman, and Kempe before them, every child abuse doctor must discover the secret world of battered children for themselves. What follows are stories from child abuse pediatricians about how and why they got into child abuse pediatrics. Many of the stories involve impactful cases that have stayed with these doctors even to this day, many involve the support of mentors in the field, all involve a deep love for the work, and the belief that this work is of profound importance to the welfare of children.

### Robert W. Block, MD, Tulsa, Oklahoma

In 1969, I was a pediatric intern at Children's Hospital of Philadelphia. A little boy came onto our service. His nose had been split with a knife, the same way it was done in the movie *Chinatown*. Back in those days, there was no easy access to foster care, so he spent some time with us. He became a sort of house staff follower. I got to know him and his situation a little bit. That was my very first case of child abuse. I can't remember much of the details but that experience plus a book by Lisa Richette titled *Throwaway Children* sparked an interest in me.

Some years later, I was working as an attending in a pediatric clinic in Oklahoma. Our social worker came to me and said that she had received a referral from child protection services for a little girl who was alleging that she'd been sexually abused. Nobody knew anything about sexual abuse as a medical diagnosis back then. I certainly didn't. She asked if I'd evaluate the girl. I said, "Well, yes, I guess I could do that." I took a history and did a physical examination. Her examination, at least to my untrained eyes at the time, was normal but she did give a compelling history of being abused.

Two weeks later, our social worker approached me again and said, "Dr. Block, you remember that little girl you saw? Well, she has a sister who is alleging that the same thing has happened to her. Would you see her?" I said, "Well, yes, I guess I could."

That night I thought, "I'm expected to know something about this, so I better read about it." The world's literature at the time was maybe a few medical articles including a couple of papers out of California by Doctor Astrid Heger.

Two weeks after that, I got a phone call from another social worker who said, "Dr. Block, I understand you're the city's expert on child sexual abuse." That's how it started.

One of the things that attracted me to the field, quite frankly, was doing something that nobody else was doing. It was very exciting. Here was something important and valuable and no one else in my area was doing it.

I love working with other disciplines. I really enjoy working with the police and child protective professionals. If you're open to their approach to a case and they're open to yours, you can get into some very interesting dialogue. It isn't just clinical medicine. We bring medical data and they bring information on the home and the family, then we collaborate in a meaningful, unique way.

### Kenneth W. Feldman, MD, Seattle, Washington

In the early 1970s, I cared for a three-year-old girl who had tap water scald burns on the top of both of her feet. We were told that she had gotten into the bathtub, turned on the water, and was scalded. It seemed to me like such an idiotic situation. A child could turn on the tap and the water would be so hot, it would almost instantly cause severe burns. This led me to review the tap water scald burns both at Harborview and at Seattle Children's. One of our clinic outreach workers and I went around the city measuring water temperatures in bathtubs. All that led to our 1978 paper (Feldman et al. 1978).

During my research, I recognized that a fair number of these children actually had sustained their injuries from abuse. I presented my results to the Ambulatory Pediatric Association. Afterward, this fellow came up to me to congratulate me on the paper. He told me how pertinent it was to his field of child abuse. He was Doctor Ray Helfer. He asked me to write a burn chapter for his book on the battered child. We kept up a fruitful mentorship over the years.

Some years later, I met that same child who had triggered my research. I was speaking at a hospital meeting about advocacy and about lobbying our state legislature to recommend water heater temperature settings to prevent these burns. These changes, by the way, cut the rate of tap water burns to a quarter of what they had been. After the meeting, this now eight-year-old child came up to me and said, "I wouldn't have been stupid enough to do that to myself. My mother's boyfriend held my feet under the hot water."

I don't think I was particularly drawn to the field at first, but after a while it clicked. Like many others, I found the work emotionally and intellectually rewarding.

### Martin Finkel, DO, Stratford, New Jersey

I came to the College of Medicine and Dentistry of New Jersey in 1979 to help found the Department of Pediatrics. Here I am at an academic institution, a new medical school with colleagues at the Robert Wood Johnson Medical School, and there was pressure to do something academic.

In the spring of 1982, the director of Medical Education asked me if I would be interested in going to hear a talk on child sexual abuse in Washington, DC. I thought to myself, "That must be a rare phenomenon." But I went anyway. After all, it was springtime in Washington.

The lecturer was Doctor Suzanne Sgroi, at the time one of the few physicians who was talking about child sexual abuse. I couldn't believe what I was hearing. I thought to myself, "I just came out of a pediatric residency program, I had a rotation in child abuse, and I never even heard child sexual abuse mentioned. If I didn't know about this issue, neither do my colleagues."

I decided then and there that, if I was going to make a difference in the field of medicine and do something academic at the same time, it was going to be in the field of child sexual abuse, where there was little literature and limited knowledge.

Two weeks later, I gave a talk to the Department of Pediatrics in my institution about what I had just heard. I had not yet even seen a sexually abused child. I basically reiterated what I learned from Doctor Sgroi. After my talk, one of the pediatricians came up to me and said, "Finkel, what's all this stuff about child sexual abuse? I've been a pediatrician for fifteen years and I've never seen a case." I said, "Precisely."

You know the old story, "If you're the only doctor in town, you're the best doctor in town?" I had no idea what I was doing but I knew

I was the best doctor for these children because I was the only doctor who was willing to see them. I reached out to child protection and law enforcement officials. They had been grappling with child sexual abuse without the help of medicine. I asked them how I could help. Soon thereafter, child welfare workers started sending children to me to evaluate.

From the very beginning, I knew I was comfortable talking to children about difficult things. I just seemed to have the temperament, the demeanor to be able to do it. I found helping children express their fears and anxieties amazingly rewarding. I think that, in order to be a child abuse doctor, besides being patient, humane, and sensitive, one has to be willing to listen to children and do so in a nonjudgmental, facilitating, and empathic manner.

I have always viewed the medical evaluation of sexual abuse as the first step in therapeutic intervention for the child. We do that by talking and listening to children. When I think about what's in the best interests of children, it's not going to be found in the prosecutorial outcome. It's going to be found in the medical and mental health outcomes. One of the things I'm most proud of has been the way the CARES (Child Abuse Research, Education and Service) Institute, where I work, has created a seamless integration of medicine and mental health.

When I sit down with a child who has found it difficult to talk about their abuse and they tell me things that they told no one else, when they demonstrate a sense of relief, as if the world has been lifted from their shoulders, it's amazing. My goal is always to create an environment to help children feel safe in sharing their stories.

This work was and is so exciting. Everything in the beginning was new. How do we visualize? How do we photograph? How do we document? How do we interpret? There were, and still are, so many exciting opportunities and challenges.

It is interesting to work with child protection, law enforcement, the courts, policy makers, legislature, and the media. I love the collegiality of working with all these other professionals.

I have been fortunate to have been one of the doctors who, along with other pioneering colleagues, contributed to the understanding of the needs of children suspected of being sexually abused. I feel that I can continue to make a difference in the community of professionals dedicated to the health and welfare of maltreated children. Every day, I feel that I can make a difference in the life of a child.

**Howard Dubowitz, MD, Baltimore, Maryland**

My interest in child abuse pediatrics started with my late dad. He was a family doctor who worked with poor blacks in Cape Town,

South Africa. He had strong values about supporting and caring for people in tough situations. He conveyed these values to me. They have been important to me all my life. When I went into medicine and then pediatrics, his values were always with me.

Around 1980, while I was a resident at Boston City Hospital, there was an incident that I have often thought was pivotal in the development of my thinking about abuse. I was working in the newborn nursery one night. I watched a mother visiting her baby and very gently playing with his foot. It struck me as a really tender moment.

The next morning, I was in our weekly "social" rounds meeting. It turned out that this mom was a heroin addict who had already lost custody of seven of her children. This new baby was scheduled to be removed from her care as well. That experience got me thinking about what was going on here. How do we think about risk to children? How do we try and protect them? How do we work with families? I thought this all sounded really interesting. I then did a two-year NIMH (National Institute of Mental Health) funded child abuse fellowship with Eli Newberger at Boston Children's Hospital.

Another memorable incident occurred very early in my fellowship. We were interviewing a family for the Boston Family Court. The family consisted of the mother, her boyfriend, and her five-year-old daughter. The question for us was whether this little girl could return home. I remember the boyfriend literally terrorizing this little girl in front of us. It was so bad that we had to intervene. My first thought was that his behavior was just hateful.

But then, in subsequent interviews, I got to know him. He told me how he had been badly abused in his home as a child, then placed in several foster homes where he was abused again. He came to have this view of the world as a rough, tough place. He had this idea that you prepared a child for this kind of world, not with hugs and kisses, but by being rough and tough with them. Not that this excused his behavior, but it's helped me understand how such behavior might develop. I often think of this man and how maltreating behavior isn't simply a matter of lousy parents who don't give a damn but often something much more complicated. I think, as professionals, when we understand the roots of behavior, it can help counter the pain and anger our work can evoke. Understanding positions us to be more helpful, more compassionate physicians.

### Alex V. Levin, MD, Philadelphia, Pennsylvania

When I was a resident in pediatrics at Children's Hospital of Philadelphia in 1983, Stephen Ludwig was my mentor. At that time, Steve was advocating for what eventually became the Ray Helfer Society. His mentorship and support, along with my own natural inclination toward social outreach, got me involved in the field.

I remember one child in particular. I actually still have a picture of him in my office. He came from a very high-risk, socially challenged family. He and his mother developed a relationship with me and, after years of working with me, she started to show pride in her son.

One day, she came in and showed me pictures of him. I thought this was real progress. This was not something she would have done in the past. The problem was that in one picture in the corner of that austere living room was a sawed-off shotgun. The next picture was of her four-year-old son holding the shotgun. Unfortunately, she didn't see that as a problem. For me, this was a moment mixed with joy and sadness, seeing her take pride in her parenting, in the successes we had made, yet knowing that the shotgun was a sign that there was a lot of work yet to be done. I can still see that family and those photographs like it was yesterday.

I've heard many times from patients and even from doctors who say, "God, how can you do this work? It's terrible!" My response has always been that child abuse pediatrics is the most rewarding work I could ever think of doing. I love this work even more than my primary specialty of pediatric ophthalmologist.

### Kent P. Hymel, MD, Hershey, Pennsylvania

In 1989, I was on active duty in the United States Air Force (USAF) medical corps assigned to Keesler Air Force Base in Biloxi, Mississippi. One week after I got there, my commander ordered me to become our local and regional medical consultant for child abuse. Ultimately, he petitioned the USAF surgeon general for me to get formal fellowship training in Colorado with Carole Jenny, a child abuse pediatrician. I could not have predicted how much I would enjoy this work. After fellowship training, I became the USAF medical consultant for child abuse.

It has been so exciting being part of the birth of a new specialty and contributing to new knowledge. I've enjoyed accomplishing some research goals that I never would have thought I could accomplish. I might well be in a position, before I retire, to have contributed something of value to our ability to more objectively make decisions about which children need a workup for abuse.

I love the challenge of the field where pediatrics sort of meets *CSI*. It's intellectually stimulating. Ideally, the detective work is balanced by advocating for children and supporting families in crisis. I believe this work best suits someone who can balance objectivity with advocacy. Being objective is the first requirement, so that you don't err in either direction. Once you've evaluated a case with an objective, systematic approach, and have diagnosed abuse, then advocacy for the child becomes the number one priority. I like the mental challenge that comes with each case being a mystery that has to be solved.

I believe the specialty needs pediatricians with a certain set of communication skills, the ability to be both empathic and professional, and the ability to establish a relationship with people under very stressful situations. Recognizing that I have the ability to be empathic and non-judgmental is precisely why I think I was meant to do this. I couldn't have known that going in. Over the years, I have come to realize that this field is exactly where I belong.

### Amanda Brownell, MD, Cincinnati, Ohio

I became interested in child abuse pediatrics after seeing several cases as a resident including one in particular in the Pediatric Intensive Care Unit. This infant girl had come in with abusive head trauma. She was not doing well. We even discussed with the family removing life support because we thought that the brain injury was so severe that she would not be able to survive. We removed her breathing tube and, surprisingly, she continued to breathe. During all of this, her father, who was the suspected perpetrator, was at her bedside participating in the decision making. It was a striking experience that sparked my desire to pursue this work.

We had this injured child. We had her father who we suspected was responsible for the injury. Yet, he was still allowed to be at her bedside. I felt it was a difficult balance, to attend to the child's needs, while also realizing that the person who had likely done this to her was standing right there, watching her struggle to breathe. This was particularly difficult for the nurses who cared for her.

The baby lived and I saw her six months later. She was with her newly adoptive mother. She had been admitted for some reason, so I went to see her. The adoptive mom was very loving toward her. She said to me, "Oh, she's saying hi. Look, look, she's saying hi." But the child just made unintelligible sounds. I don't think she was actually saying hi since her abuse had left her blind, deaf, and with significant deficits. I suppose being adopted by a loving family was some consolation. (Author's note: This child's story, about Angel, is further discussed in Chapter 9.)

One of the things I have thought about this work is that you are helping children who you will never meet. I may not be able to save a child who is dying in the intensive care unit, but I can save their siblings by advocating for their removal from an unsafe home. They may have a chance for a happier life because of my advocacy, even though I will never meet them.

**Christine Barron, MD, Providence, Rhode Island**

When I was a pediatric resident at Brown, I was expected to spend a month in the child abuse clinic. I had heard from other residents how depressing it was. I thought, "How am I going to manage thirty days of hearing all these horrible stories?" I was planning on becoming a pediatric emergency physician. But then I thought, "You know what? I'm just going to go and learn what I can, so that when I see a case of abuse in the emergency department I'll know what to do."

After the first week of the rotation, my husband told me, "You're going to do this for a career." Shocked I replied, "No I'm not! I'm doing emergency medicine. What do you mean?" He could see how much I enjoyed the clinical puzzles, going through all the evidence, working with medical and nonmedical professionals, trying to figure out what happened. He told me, "This is the sort of field that chooses you and I believe you have been chosen."

Carole Jenny had just started two months earlier as director of our new child protection program. By the end of the rotation, she said to me. "I think you should do this." I thought about it for a while then I told her, "You know what? I think you're right."

After residency, I completed a two-year fellowship with Carole at Brown and then I started a program in Worcester, Massachusetts. It was quite a challenge. When I started, police and child protective service workers were not talking to each other. I was told that was the way it was and I would be unable to change it. I thought, "I'm going to try and get everyone to sit down together and talk. If it doesn't work, it doesn't work." But it did work. It was so successful that Lieutenant Governor Healey, under then Massachusetts governor Mitt Romney, heard about what we were doing and came to one of our meetings. He wanted to learn how to implement this type of program throughout Massachusetts.

After leaving Worcester to return to the child protection program in Providence, I looked back at what we had accomplished in Worcester County. I was a young physician and had started a program that still exists today. I think it is amazing to work in a field like child abuse where our contributions can have such an impact. Despite all the challenges, thinking about that keeps me going.

Now 16 years later, I still love the work. People ask me all the time, "What do you do for work?" When I say I am a pediatrician, they respond positively and ask me questions about their child's health. That's when I say "I'm not that kind of pediatrician. I specialize in child abuse." Then they say, "Oh my god, how horrible." I have even

heard that from pediatric oncologists, which is ironic, since I could never do their work.

I always look at the work as a balance of sorts. I see children who have been abused and who I can help protect and I see children who were not abused and I can protect them from being removed from their homes. I love the balance.

My father, who has since passed away, was a New York City firefighter. In the eloquent way of a firefighter, his mandate to all of his children was that, whatever we chose to do with our lives, we had to always remember two things. We had to make the world a better place than it was when we came into it and we had to always remember that we came from blue-collar stock. We should strive to help those less fortunate than us. I think I would have made him proud.

### Henry Kempe, MD (deceased), Denver, Colorado

It seems fitting to include here the words of Henry Kempe in a letter dated October 29, 1983 (Heins 1984, 3296). "My involvement in child abuse was at first far from humane: it was candidly intellectual at least at part. Day after day, while making rounds at the University of Colorado Medical School whose department of pediatrics I headed since 1956, I was shown children with diagnoses by residents and by consultants and attending physicians which simply were examples of either ignorance or denial. I thought very much the latter. I was shown children who had thrived for seven months and then developed 'spontaneous subdural hematomas,' 'multiple bruises of unknown etiology' in children who had no bleeding disorders, 'Osteogenesis Imperfecta Tarda' in children who had normal bones by x-ray except that they showed many healing fractures, 'impetigo' in children with skin lesions which were clearly inflicted, 'accidental burns of buttocks' in symmetrical form which could only occur from dunking a child who had soiled into a bucket of hot water. We did often learn from one or both parents in time and with patient and kindly approaches that these were all inflicted injuries."

Finally, in his seminal article on the battered child syndrome, Kempe wrote, "The battered child syndrome, a clinical condition in young children who have received serious physical abuse, is a frequent cause of permanent injury or death. The syndrome should be considered in any child exhibiting evidence of fracture of any bone, subdural hematoma, failure to thrive, soft tissue swellings or skin bruising. To the informed physician, the bones tell a story the child is too young or too frightened to tell" (Kempe et al. 1962, 18).

## About Three Children

Throughout my medical career, I have been interested in family violence. It is difficult for me to understand or explain why. Perhaps this interest stems from growing up in a violent inner-city South Philadelphia neighborhood where the sounds of gunshots, fighting, and police sirens were all too common. I did not, however, grow up in a violent home. Yet, early childhood experiences, good or bad, remembered or forgotten, have a profound impact on the direction our lives take.

As a pediatric resident, what little I saw of abuse mystified me. My first case, in 1974, was an infant with an unexplained subdural hematoma, a blood clot covering the surface of his brain. Today, such a finding would beg the question, was this child abused? Such a finding would likely now lead to a comprehensive abuse workup, ideally performed by a board-certified child abuse pediatrician. The workup would include a careful physical examination, x-rays, other studies to look for alternative medical explanations, a careful assessment of the social history, and involvement of the child welfare and law enforcement communities. Often, such a detailed assessment would reveal other evidence to support a diagnosis of abuse, evidence such as old fractures, bruises, sometimes siblings who have been abused, and significant family risk factors such as domestic violence and substance abuse.

But in 1974, much of the diagnostic discussion of my case focused not on abuse but on obscure and unlikely alternative explanations for the blood. This was not bad medicine, just medicine as practiced in its time. Unfortunately, because abuse was not considered much less diagnosed in 1974, this infant was sent home only to return later, even more badly injured.

For the next several years, I saw the occasional abuse case, first as a pediatric resident, then as a practicing pediatrician, then as an emergency medicine resident, and then as a practicing emergency physician. However, nothing prepared me for the two children I would see one Sunday morning in 1984.

A badly beaten five-year-old girl and her equally beaten two-year-old brother were brought to my emergency room by a child protective worker. The story, offered by the parents, was that the children had fallen down a flight of stairs.

After examining the obviously abused children, I took photographs of their injuries with my Canon 35mm SLR camera, a camera I carried with me everywhere. I have always loved photography and secretly hoped that this love would serve me in some professional fashion. Little did I know that my attempts to emulate famous photographers such as Edward Weston and Dorothea Lange would translate into the art and science of child abuse photo-documentation.

As I look now at the faded Ektachrome slides of these two children, I can vividly remember them. One slide shows the five-year-old with a thin smile and a mask of bright red bruises circling bloodshot eyes; another slide shows extensive bruising over the entire left side of her face, perhaps from blows by a right-handed perpetrator. Still another shows her upper chest where two large thumb-size bruises bracket her lower neck. Only the wrists are visible on the single image that remains of her brother, wrists badly bruised, abraded, and scarred in a pattern that could only have been caused by being tied up. Clearly, the bruises, scars, and abrasions on these children could not have been from a single or even multiple falls.

I wrote a report detailing all the injuries stating my opinion that these children had been abused and were not safe returning to the home where the abuse occurred. I left the children in the hands of the child protective worker and went on to my next patient. I expected that would be the end of it, unless I had to testify in court.

Some months later, I was surprised to find my name in a local newspaper article describing a successful plea bargain in my case. The district attorney described in some detail how impressed he was with my report and how that report had been instrumental in obtaining the guilty plea.

My meticulous attention to that abuse case and others eventually reached the supervisory level of Child Protective Services (CPS) in Maine. A short time later, again on a Sunday morning, a child protective supervisor called to ask me if I would see a four-month-old girl who had just been admitted to the hospital. The baby's father had found her unresponsive and had called 911. When a paramedic went to clear her airway, he found an infant's sock wedged deep in her throat. The paramedic removed the sock and saved her life. I still have a photo of that folded, bloody sock. Clearly, someone had jammed the sock down her throat, perhaps to silence her crying.

The call to me from CPS though had less to do with the obvious attempt to silence the baby than with an injury she had sustained two months earlier. Her father had taken her to the emergency department because she was not using her right arm. He told the medical staff that he was giving her a bath the night before and she had slipped from the side of the tub. As she fell, he had grabbed her by the arm and now she was not moving it. X-rays showed a fracture of the upper arm bone, the humerus, an injury we now know to be highly suspicious for abuse in a child that young. The infant was seen by an orthopedic surgeon who described in his report how he had considered child abuse, but that, after careful, detailed, and repeated questioning of the father, he felt comfortable with the father's story of an accident, and comfortable not reporting the injury to CPS. The surgeon sent them on their way. Now, two months later, this same infant was back in the emergency department after almost suffocating to death.

I drove to the hospital, saw the now successfully resuscitated infant, and reviewed the x-rays from two months earlier. Looking at those x-rays was a revelation, in part because of the potentially horrific consequences of the mistake that had been made, but, even more so, because of the nature of the mistake. An important component of the fracture had been missed by the orthopedist, by the emergency room doctor, and by the radiologist. Even I, at that time relatively new to the field of child abuse, could see that the fracture showed signs of healing. This baby had not stopped using her arm that day. She likely had stopped using the arm at least two weeks earlier, putting the lie to her father's story of an injury the night before. Given the two injuries, both apparently occurring while in the care of the father, it was clear that this child was not safe in that home.

I wish I could tell you the ultimate outcome for these three children. As with many children, what happens after a medical diagnosis of abuse is hidden deep in the sometimes impenetrable offices of the child welfare and criminal justice systems and sometimes inside the equally impenetrable homes of abusive families.

Still, I made diagnoses that, at least in the short term, helped save three children from further abuse. That gratification, that sense of being uniquely useful, spurred me toward a career in child abuse pediatrics. This was a field that moved me intellectually and emotionally, that exposed me to the secret heart of family life. Even now, after 30 years of seeing children who have been abused and children who have not, I know that each family will be unique and that each story, if listened to carefully, will be sometimes sad, sometimes tragic, sometimes hopeful, sometimes even joyful, but always intriguing.

As told in the aforementioned child abuse pediatrician stories, what was happening to me in Maine was also happening to many of my medical colleagues around the country. Doctors, who took an interest in abuse, were sought out by child welfare professionals and asked to examine children. A cadre of such doctors began to gather at national pediatric meetings and talk about cases, protocols, and procedures. It was the beginning of a new specialty. At first, we called it forensic pediatrics. In 2006, the American Board of Pediatrics formally recognized the new specialty and called it child abuse pediatrics.

Thus, the story of child abuse pediatrics as a medical specialty in the United States advanced in fits and starts from Ambroise Tardieu in 1860 to Henry Kempe in 1962 to the Helfer Society in 1999 and finally to a Board of Pediatrics recognized specialty in 2006. One would have thought that all the groundwork had been laid for a successful specialty. It had not. There was still much to learn, particularly about how to avoid mistakes that put children at risk of further abuse, even death.

## CHAPTER TWO

# Mistakes: It Could Be Anyone

There are two types of mistakes a physician can make when diagnosing child abuse. One is overdiagnosis, saying abuse has occurred when it has not. The other is underdiagnosis, saying abuse has not occurred when it has. Both types of mistakes or diagnostic errors can have serious consequences for children and families. Saying a child has been abused when they have not may result in a child being removed from an innocent family. Saying a child has not been abused when they have can lead to further injury, even death.

In the medical literature, by far the more common error is underdiagnosis. In 1999, a paper was published by Carole Jenny and her colleagues at the University of Colorado on missed cases of abusive head trauma (Jenny et al. 1999). The authors noted that the impetus for the paper was a 1995 case of a 14-month-old infant with abusive head trauma whom they evaluated. Before he was presented to them at their hospital with multiple old and new fractures and permanent brain injury, he had been examined by other medical providers a total of seven times. Each time, the diagnosis of child abuse had been missed and the child had gone home to suffer further injury.

In their review of cases of abusive head trauma at their institution, the authors identified 54 abused infants whose diagnosis of child abuse had been missed by medical providers. Fifty-four misdiagnosed infants, out of a total of 173, represent an astounding 30 percent underdiagnosis rate. Fifteen of these 54 children were further injured after the initial missed diagnosis and, of these, five died.

Jenny and her colleagues found that signs of abuse were more likely to be missed if the child was white, rather than of minority race, and from an intact family, rather than one where the parents were separated. Clearly, these results raised the issue of bias, in these cases, the bias of assuming a white child from an intact home could not be a victim of abuse.

A number of papers have further discussed the issue of physician bias (Croskerry 2002; Croskerry 2003; Dawson and Arkes 1987; Laskey 2014; Skellern 2015). What are some of these biases? Why do physicians make these mistakes?

In nontechnical terms, some of these biases include jumping to conclusions, not waiting for all the data to come in, ignoring conflicting data, stereotyping individuals as good or bad, and failing to appreciate that common things happen commonly. Some have fancy names that don't necessarily convey their meaning but, once understood, the nature and cause of these biases are all too obvious.

Anchoring is the tendency to prematurely lock onto a diagnosis and then fail to consider new information in conflict with that diagnosis. This is similar to confirmation bias, where the provider accepts only information that confirms what they believe and rejects conflicting data. I once saw an infant with a broken leg who I was certain was abused. The child protective worker thought the break happened from an accidental fall even though no history of a fall was forthcoming from the parents. She wanted to send the child home with her parents even before I had x-rayed the rest of the body. With some difficulty and only after a call to her supervisor, I convinced her to wait. Subsequent x-rays showed additional fractures. Even with that, the worker still thought it was all an accident and wanted to send the child home with her parents. It was as if she were stuck, anchored to her original decision. Luckily, the child did not go home with those parents.

Availability bias occurs when a provider makes a diagnosis not based on the unique circumstances of the case at hand but based on a diagnosis that readily comes to mind. Prior experience rather than the circumstances of the current case can influence decision making. Because most providers rarely see serious child abuse, they often mistake it for something else. I have frequently seen children with bruising where the primary care provider decided it was more likely to be a coagulation disorder, despite the fact that abusive bruising is far more common than a bleeding disorder. In at least a few of these cases, while the physician waited for the results of the bleeding tests, the child was killed.

Outcome bias happens when a provider opts for the diagnosis that will lead to a good (translate happy) outcome. The clinician offers the diagnosis they hope for rather than the one that is correct. Affective bias is similar. In these cases, the provider draws conclusions that avoid an unpleasant task, such as talking to a family about abuse. Once, following a case discussion, a medical student told me she felt bad that the diagnosis was abuse. She had not wanted that. I expressed some sympathy for her emotional difficulty but told her that our job is not to find the diagnosis we want. Our job was to find the diagnosis that is correct.

Confirmation bias is the tendency to only look for evidence that supports a particular diagnosis rather than evidence that refutes it. An example is using insensitive indicators such as parental behavior or parent-child interaction as an indication that abuse has not occurred. Primary care providers often say that they "know" the family and "know" that they could not have abused the child, despite only having had limited contact with the family in a controlled office environment.

I also see this frequently in family members who tell me that their partner, their son, their daughter-in-law, for example, could not have abused the child because they "know" them. My response is always that they might know what they themselves did or didn't do, but they really don't know anyone else well enough to know with any certainty that they couldn't abuse a child.

Feedback bias occurs when we do not get immediate feedback about the accuracy of our diagnoses. If we miss a child abuse diagnosis and never learn about it, we are likely to make the same mistake again. This kind of bias is ubiquitous in our field where families disappear never to return, and where the child welfare system does not talk to providers about the outcome of a case. We never know if abuse was substantiated, much less, if it later reoccurred. We never know if we were right saying a child had not been abused unless we have the terrible experience of later reading about a death in the newspaper. When I asked the child abuse pediatricians I interviewed for this book if they had ever made a mistake, several acknowledged that this was a problem in our field. How would they know if they made a mistake if they never hear back about what happened after their evaluation?

Visceral bias is using one's gut to judge a family. This is similar to attribution bias where one uses negative or positive stereotyping. Many of us have an image in our heads about what an abuser looks like. If the parent does not fit that image, we then decide that they could not be an abuser. I have often heard professionals dismiss allegations of abuse because "these are good parents." Those of us in the field know that there is no profile of what an abuser does or does not look like.

Laskey (2014) noted that there are a number of incorrect assumptions made by professionals in child abuse assessments, which could lead to error. They assume that caretakers will tell the truth about what happened to the child. They think they know their patients' families and can judge whether someone is an abuser. Finally, they believe that they can judge from a child's interaction with their parent whether that child has been abused.

Laskey also suggested that errors or biases can be prevented by avoiding premature closure (prematurely stopping the assessment before all the data is in), by seeking objective information from all sources, and by working within a multidisciplinary team.

Flaherty and her colleagues have looked at the problem through a different lens (Flaherty and Fingarson 2012; Flaherty and Sege 2005). They broke the problem down to failure to diagnose child abuse and failure to report once child abuse is diagnosed. The former occurs for a number of reasons including insufficient data collection, bias including racial and socioeconomic bias, psychological barriers, and a lack of knowledge and training. The latter occurs because of physician uncertainty, unfamiliarity with child protective services, previous unpleasant experiences with child protective services not helping the family, unwillingness to "hurt" their relationship with the family, and fear of the legal system, particularly court.

There are many more types of biases and thinking errors in the medical literature. In some cases, these biases and errors have minimal consequences, for example, treating an ear infection with an unnecessary antibiotic to avoid a lengthy and uncomfortable discussion with a parent who insists on an antibiotic. In child abuse, however, the consequences can be dire indeed.

What then is the solution to this problem apart from education and experience? In at least two studies, a board-certified child abuse pediatrician, who sees hundreds, if not thousands, of children for abuse assessment, who often works with a team, and who is intimately familiar with the literature on child abuse and on thinking errors and biases, is far better at making the correct diagnosis than a general physician who might see a couple of abuse cases a year, if that.

Anderst and colleagues (2009) reviewed children who were reported to child protective services for suspected physical abuse. All were evaluated first by a general pediatrician, family or emergency doctor, then later by a child abuse pediatrician. In 115 children, primary care doctors offered a diagnosis of abuse or not abuse, but on review by a child abuse pediatrician, 49 of these children had their diagnosis changed. In 80 percent of these 49, the diagnosis was changed from abuse to not abuse, saving families from unnecessary intervention. In the remaining 20 percent, the diagnosis was changed from not abuse to abuse, protecting children from further harm.

In a paper by McGuire and colleagues (McGuire, Martin, and Leventhal 2011), 187 children referred to child protective services were compared in terms of diagnosis made by child abuse doctors versus primary care providers (pediatricians, family doctors, emergency physicians).

The two child abuse pediatricians who reviewed each case independently were strongly in agreement with each other. Almost 50 percent of children were diagnosed as definitely or probably abused, while 8 percent were diagnosed as uncertain, and 43 percent as probably not abused.

However, child abuse pediatricians disagreed with the primary care provider in almost 50 percent of cases and disagreed with the child protective worker in almost 40 percent of cases. Remarkably, the child abuse pediatrician was far more likely to rate a case as not abuse compared to the primary care physician and the child protective worker who rated it as abuse. In other words, both the primary care physician and the child protective worker tended to overdiagnose abuse compared to the child abuse expert. In almost 30 percent of cases, where the expert thought abuse had not happened and child protective services and the primary physician thought it had, the child had already been removed from the home.

Those who would vilify child abuse pediatricians as hired agents of the state, as always finding abuse even when it didn't happen, should read these papers. It might be reasonably concluded from these studies that every child in the United States suspected of being abused should be evaluated by a board-certified child abuse pediatrician.

---

There is the potential for deep, unremitting pain in child abuse work when getting a diagnosis wrong, particularly in failing to protect a vulnerable child who then goes on to be further harmed or even killed. At issue is not whether this happens, but whether we learn from these cases and how these experiences shape us.

**Kent P. Hymel, MD, Hershey, Pennsylvania**

I think that each of us has made a few mistakes. The children who resonate the most with me are those that I recognized in hindsight had been abused. Yet, at the time I didn't consider it because I hadn't done my training. I can think of two or three children I saw, before I became a child abuse pediatrician, where I missed the diagnosis. Those are the ones that haunt me.

In 1985, I was called to the emergency department to see an eight-month-old child who was vomiting. I examined the child. I documented the vital signs. I documented a normal abdomen examination. I documented that there was no diarrhea and no sick contact at home.

I even documented that there were no signs of skin trauma. I've always been very compulsive about my documentation.

I gave the parents instructions about watching for signs of dehydration, going from clear liquids to foods, watching for diarrhea, and to come back as needed. The next morning, when I came in to work, I was told that this child had come back to the emergency room. They had just completed a code (cardiac arrest resuscitation attempt) that had failed. The child was dead. The autopsy revealed that the child had died from a liver laceration, a blow or blows to the abdomen. Of course, the family never said anything to me about possible abdominal trauma. I didn't specifically recall asking about it though. In other words, child abuse never crossed my mind.

I looked back at my notes. Because the child died, it was reviewed by others in my department. The one thing I failed to recognize at the time was there was some tachycardia (rapid heartbeat) that I attributed it to the child being unhappy with my examination. The child's pulse pressure (possible sign of shock) was also narrow. I blamed myself for not recognizing these early signs of shock. So the parents took him home, put him to bed, and then he slowly bled to death from his liver injury. By the time they went to wake him in the morning, it was too late.

I fault myself for not paying more attention to the fact that the child had been vomiting without diarrhea. Now I know to consider not only abdominal trauma but head trauma. Could I have done more? I didn't document looking at the retina. Now, if I have vomiting without diarrhea, I will do that.

There are lots of excuses I could have made about why I missed the diagnosis. I don't accept any of them. That child still haunts me. I still have a visual image of that child in my head. I failed him.

### Kenneth W. Feldman, MD, Seattle, Washington

One very memorable case was a toddler who had what is known as a "toddler" fracture of the tibia (a minor, usually accidental, fracture of the shin bone in a two- or three-year-old caused by a twisting fall, for example, from jumping off of a couch). He also had a skull fracture, which gave me pause. Yet, both injuries had fairly plausible explanations, that is to say, the accidental explanations being offered by the mother seemed to explain the two separate injuries. I had been consulted by child protective services to review the records. I never saw the child.

After the review, I told CPS, "You know, these sound like pretty legitimate accidental causes for these injuries, but I'm really worried about everything else that's said about the mother." There were lots of social concerns about parenting and drug use. Unfortunately, I think child protective services heard the former but not the latter. This child was eventually killed by his mother. I don't recall the specific details of the death, but he did die from inflicted trauma.

There was another child who I still wonder about. He had several fractures while in the parents' care. He had no evidence of a metabolic bone disorder (such as osteogenesis imperfecta often called "brittle bone disease") to account for the fractures. I diagnosed abuse and he went into foster care. But there, he had more fractures with minimal trauma. Because of this, I wondered if his original fractures might have been from some rare, unidentified bone disorder. Lab work failed to identify any inherited diseases of fragile bones, but I withdrew my original diagnosis of abuse and he was returned to his parents.

### Alex V. Levin, MD, MHSc, FRCSC, FAAO, Philadelphia, Pennsylvania

I don't remember the details of the case, just the outcome, and how it made me feel, then and even now. A baby was admitted with a subdural hematoma (bleeding on the surface of the brain from an injury) and the team, including a child abuse pediatrician, neurosurgeon, and myself as the pediatric ophthalmologist, thought the head injury was from an accidental fall. Later, the same child came back to the hospital dead from abuse.

What do you say? What do you do? We made a mistake. Afterward, we racked our brains trying to figure out how we had missed it. We asked ourselves a thousand questions. Were we too dismissive of abuse or too accepting of the differential diagnosis we always consider? To this day, I feel like we had blood on our hands.

### John McCann, MD, Davis, California

Early in my medical career, I remember being asked by my nurse if I would be willing to examine a girl whose mother said her daughter had an injury to her "private parts."

My colleague, Dr. Shirley Anderson (an early pioneer in the medical assessment of sexual abuse), who usually saw these children, wasn't there that day. I said, "Oh sure." Of course at that time I had very little experience evaluating prepubertal girls' genitalia, particularly one with an injury.

Even at such an early stage in my career, I could see that she had what appeared to be a relatively minor genital injury. Her mother had described a fall and I concluded that that was not an unreasonable explanation, but that I would like to have her reexamined by Dr. Anderson.

As I pulled out of our parking lot on my way to lunch, I remember seeing this mother and her daughter leaving our office. They both were walking down the sidewalk, the daughter several feet behind her mother. Both of them had their heads down looking at the sidewalk. We never saw them again.

The nursing staff tried several times to track them down but the telephone number the mother had given us didn't exist and the address she had given us was a parking lot. This being the "pre-child protective service" era, we never did find them. To this day, I'm sure this was my first, although unrecognized, case of child sexual abuse.

### Richard D. Krugman, MD, Aurora, Colorado

There was an eight-year-old boy who was riding his bike in Aspen on a beautiful June night. He was going down the Rio Grande Trail. He left at five o'clock. His parents told him to come home at six for dinner, but he didn't get home until eight o'clock. It was unusual for him to be so late. When he finally came home, he was pale and mute. He wouldn't say a word. His parents took him to the emergency room where he was examined. Drug tests were performed among other things and he was kept overnight. The next day he still would not talk. His doctors didn't know what was going on, so they had the parents drive him down to Glenwood Springs where there was a pediatric neurologist who did an EEG and a head CT. Both were normal. He still would not talk.

He was then sent to Grand Junction where he was seen by another neurologist who ordered a head MRI, which was also normal. He was then sent to Denver where he saw three more pediatric neurologists who, after a week of testing, decided that he had a psychiatric problem. So then he was admitted to a residential mental health treatment facility.

Three months into his stay, he started to talk about what had happened to him while on his bike ride. He told the doctors that he was pulled off the bike, a knife was held to his throat and he was anally raped. Nobody in Aspen, Glenwood, Grand Junction, or Denver had looked at his anus. If they had looked at his anus that first night, they would have likely seen that he had been sodomized. When I teach medical students and residents about this case, I say to them, "You can't not look."

### Allison M. Jackson, MD, MPH, Washington, D.C.

I once saw a burned infant. The team and I thought the burns could have occurred accidentally while dad was bathing the infant. We found

no other injuries, but sometime later the same infant presented to another facility with new concerns, was evaluated by another child abuse pediatrician, and was found to have multiple inflicted fractures. I don't know if it was "group think" but obviously we were wrong about the burn.

I couldn't stop wondering, "How could I have missed that?" But then I realized that we are all human, not psychic. Those injuries looked accidental to me. There are injuries where an accidental explanation is possible and could fit the injury pattern but the accidental explanation is not true. A parent or caretaker could give a solid sounding accidental explanation that is simply a lie. Knowing that the baby had suffered additional injuries after I had laid hands on them was very disturbing and troubling. It taught me to be sympathetic to other medical professionals, less informed than I about child abuse, who make a mistake.

I once evaluated a case where an infant was killed by a daycare provider. Some days earlier, his parents had taken him to their pediatrician for bruises. The pediatrician worked the baby up for a coagulation disorder and apparently never considered abuse, perhaps because the parents didn't fit the profile of a child abuser. But they weren't the abuser! The baby later died from multiple injuries inflicted by the daycare provider.

Every time I get a case like that, it strengthens my resolve to continue the work, to educate other professionals to not make that kind of mistake. This baby didn't have a bleeding disorder, he was being tortured.

Even worse, in this case, I knew the pediatrician. I never talked to her about what had happened. I didn't want to make it any worse for her. I'm sure she realized the terrible mistake she made. I'm sure it plagues her. I can only imagine because I know how I felt about my case and that was not even a fatality.

### Lynn K. Sheets, MD, Milwaukee, Wisconsin

There is one that will haunt me forever. I saw a four-week-old with a skull fracture. I could not determine if it was abuse or possibly a birth injury. Though not routine at the time, I did recommend a second set of x-rays of the entire body in two weeks. The initial set had been otherwise negative (in cases of possible physical abuse of infants, sometimes the initial set of whole body x-rays are negative for additional fractures, while a follow-up set in two weeks will show evidence of healing fractures that could not be seen on the initial set). I made the recommendation for the second set but for some reason they were not done.

The baby came back six weeks later with a fatal inflicted abdominal injury. For me, that was a game changer. Ever since then, I have made absolutely sure that every follow-up x-ray I recommend gets done. We now have 100 percent compliance with that. We don't miss follow-up skeletal surveys anymore.

Another case was that of a two-month-old boy with what we would later call a "sentinel injury." I keep the photos of this little guy for teaching. We had been aware that often, when a child came in to the hospital with serious physical abuse, the parent would also give a history of prior injury that had not been investigated.

Two days before we saw him, a visiting nurse had gone to the home and seen a cheek bruise. The nurse accepted the mother's explanation that a two-year-old sibling had hit him with a Barbie doll. Two days later he came to us with severe head trauma, a healing femur fracture, and healing rib fractures. He still had the bruise. If only the nurse had not accepted the story, if only he had been seen by us two days earlier, we would have done a skeletal survey that would have demonstrated the healing fractures, this boy would be normal now rather than severely brain damaged. After that case and so many like it before, I thought, "This had got to stop." I started thinking about a study we could do. The end result was our sentinel injury study that was finally published in 2013.

I still think about that little boy. If only we could have done the sentinel injury study sooner, maybe he would be normal today. Had I pursued the study sooner and teaching about sentinel injuries, the way we do now, I think that child and others like him would have been spared. And that's on me. I have to deal with that. It's on me.

(In 2013, Sheets and colleagues [2013] from the Medical College of Wisconsin published a paper on what they called "Sentinel Injuries." They defined a sentinel injury as any injury visible to at least one parent before more serious subsequent abuse led to hospitalization. Examples they offered included bruising, mouth injuries, and minor burns in infants. In an analysis comparing abused with non-abused children, they found that 27 percent of abused infants had a history of previous sentinel injury, while none of 101 non-abused infants acting as controls had a previous sentinel injury. Sentinel injuries occurred in early infancy usually before three months of age. Medical providers were aware of these injuries and did not intervene in 40 percent of these children. Many child abuse pediatricians feel that because of this paper, countless children had been saved from further abuse, even death.)

## About David

In 1988, I left emergency medicine and embarked on a career in child abuse pediatrics. It was an exciting time. Like-minded colleagues and I would meet at pediatric conferences around the country to discuss the latest developments in our emerging specialty. New papers were coming out, at first occasionally, then in a flood. There were new assessment techniques, new protocols, and new colleagues. We were a young specialty, not yet fully recognized. Even so, we all felt a passion for the work, the multidisciplinary collaboration, and the exciting new ideas. It was a time full of promise—until I saw David.

David was six months old when he came with his parents to see me. He was referred by his pediatrician because of a broken leg. An x-ray had revealed a fracture of the lower end of the femur (thigh bone). It was a fairly minor fracture. Still, any fracture is concerning for abuse in a six-month-old and this fracture was unexplained. According to the parents, no accident had happened.

His parents were middle-class professionals. Both presented well, that is to say, they were well dressed, engaging, and forthright in answering my questions. I felt comfortable with them. I even knew David's mother as a professional colleague. David's dad showed up at my office in a jacket and tie. He was not angry or upset. He openly and easily answered all of my questions. He thought the fracture might have happened when he was holding David under the arms and playfully bouncing him up and down on his knee. This mechanism, where the leg is straight and the force applied to the foot is transmitted to the upper leg, is possibly the kind of mechanism that might cause this injury. I remember worrying about the injury, but I was swayed by the parents' presentation. I accepted the explanation, and they left.

After I saw David, I spoke to his pediatrician. She had no other concerns about the family. David had come in for all of his checkups and shots. There was no other history of injury or other reason to worry about the parents. We agreed that although an unexplained, or in this case tentatively explained, fracture in a six-month-old was worrisome, the explanation offered by the father was plausible and the general presentation of the family was not in the least concerning.

Twice in my career I have been told news that made me feel like I had been viciously kicked in the stomach. In both cases, the news was that a child who I had evaluated for abuse had subsequently died. This was the first of those cases.

A month later, I was sitting in my office when the phone rang. Even now, 30 years later, I can remember that call and how it made me feel. The call was from a nurse in our emergency department telling me that David had come into the hospital not breathing and that every attempt to resuscitate him had failed. He had died. The rest of the conversation was a blur.

The history, as she told me, was vague; something about dad finding the baby not breathing. I knew that was not what happened. I knew what the medical examiner would find even before she performed the autopsy. I went to the autopsy anyway to see what I already knew, that David had sustained a fatal inflicted head injury. I knew that David had been killed by his father, even before he confessed to the police that he had slammed the baby's head down on the floor in a rage.

As I walked out of the medical examiner's office after the autopsy, I remember feeling very alone, very sad. I couldn't stop crying.

In his confession, David's father said that he had become frustrated with his son's crying and had shaken him then slammed his head down the floor. There was no trial. He pled guilty and was sent to prison. The sentence was not long, as I recall.

I spoke again to the baby's pediatrician who was as mystified as I that this had happened in this particular family. I asked the father's attorney after David's father went to prison if I could meet with him so that I could try to understand why and how this had happened. I was particularly interested in learning if the broken leg was indeed an accident. My suspicion was that the mechanism he described to me, bouncing the child on his leg, was what had happened, but what he did not tell me was that he was frustrated, maybe even angry, while bouncing David and was using inappropriate, excessive force. But at the time he did not tell me that. I suspect he was afraid of the potential criminal repercussions. If he had told me the truth, there would have been law enforcement and child protective investigations. He would have had to leave the home. His marriage would have likely ended. Maybe he would have gone to prison, maybe not, but the outcome for David would have been so very different. After his conviction and imprisonment, he refused to speak with me. I could never learn the truth about the broken leg.

For days after the autopsy, I couldn't stop crying and for months afterward I questioned my competency and my career choice. Somehow I persevered. I talked to colleagues around the country, many of whom were sympathetic and interested in hearing me talk about how I felt.

It would be true but too facile to say that I was not the one who had killed David. It would be true but too facile to say that I had been lied to, that the father did not tell me how frustrated and angry he was when he bounced David up and down and broke the leg. It is the nature of child abuse that perpetrators lie. I should have recognized that. What stopped me? I suspect that it was the middle-class professional facing me, someone just like me.

Some months later, after the plea bargain and imprisonment of David's father, his mother and I met in my office after everyone else had gone home. I don't remember who asked for the meeting. I remember how quiet the office was. I had been anxious about the meeting, not knowing what she would say or even what I might say. Would she be angry with me? Certainly I was angry with myself. Would she feel blamed by me? I did not blame her for failing to see the risk her husband posed to her son. Much, though not all, abuse happens in secret. Sometimes there are clues, unexplained bruises in an infant, domestic violence, substance abuse, anger by the perpetrator at the baby for crying, even horrible name calling. I did not think any of these clues were present in this case. Yet, I knew some of her coworkers and friends blamed her for not seeing the signs. After all, she was an educated professional.

When we met, there were no recriminations or blame, no anger. There was deep sadness and many tears on both our parts. I think we both felt ashamed and angry, her more than me, since there was now this horrible absence in her life, this unimaginable grief. The meeting ended up being more for my benefit than hers and it did help me decide to continue to do the work that I loved.

David's death was preventable and there were lessons to be learned. In particular, amidst the agony of my failure to protect David, I relearned a terrible truth about human existence. I had always known, from growing up in a violent inner city, that life was inherently unpredictable, that trust was fleeting, and that safety was an illusion. But somehow, in the ensuing years of medical school, of residency and practice in mostly safe environments, I had forgotten all of that.

I also had suffered from the illusion that parents will usually tell the truth, and that if they didn't, I would be able to look into the eye and see that they were lying.

This case burned away any naive illusions I might have had about the ways of the world, about abusive parents, and about my own investigative skills. I no longer try to divine whether someone is telling me the truth or not. I realized that I can never know the answer to these questions by just looking at parents. The only thing I can ever truly know is the condition of the child, the nature of the injuries, and what those injuries tell me about what happened to that child.

Some might find that this uncertainty drives them away from the work. Rather than drive me away, this realization spurred me on to continue the work with even greater commitment. It was as if I had come home again to the violently unpredictable world of my childhood in inner-city Philadelphia.

Individual case experiences often determine how a doctor practices. This was true for me after David died. I would never again take a parent at his or her word. I would never again assume that an injury was accidental without a thorough investigation. Since David's death, the guiding principle of my career has been "if I am going to err, it will be on the side of child safety." Ideally, it would be best to not make a mistake at all. But if I have to make a mistake, it will be to never send a child back to an abusive home to be further abused, if not killed. That for me was the lesson of David's death.

Although I took to heart this lesson after David died, it was inevitable, given the nature of the work, that I would make another mistake. This time, I was simply outwitted.

CHAPTER THREE

# Down the Rabbit Hole with Baron Munchausen

## About Nevaeh

I saw three-month-old Nevaeh only once when she was alive. She had been hospitalized several times during her short life. Her mother kept bringing her in because she said Nevaeh had suddenly stopped breathing, turned blue, and went limp at home. Each time she came into the hospital, she was fine.

Such events can happen. For example, a child might reflux stomach contents, choke, and turn blue. These episodes are usually benign but extremely frightening to parents. Many times no explanation is found and ultimately the symptoms go away. Events like this were originally called ALTE or Acute Life Threatening Events. Most recently, to emphasize their generally benign nature, the name was changed to BRUE or Brief Resolved Unexplained Events.

In Nevaeh's case, no cause was ever found. Yet, her symptoms did not go away. Oddly, despite her having been in the hospital several times, these spells had only been witnessed by her mother and only at home. During her brief life, she had spent as many days in the hospital as at home. She never had a spell in the hospital.

After multiple hospitalizations with no evidence of any cause for the spells and no spells in the hospital, despite the mother presenting as caring and competent, the medical staff grew concerned that maybe Nevaeh's mother was making it all up, perhaps for attention. They asked me to see her.

My examination of Nevaeh, my review of the medical records, and my interview of her mother yielded no specific clues. Her mother was appropriate with me and attentive to her infant daughter.

As I tried to decide whether to wait and see what would happen next time, or go out on a limb and recommend Nevaeh be removed from her mother's care, one of the resident doctor told me they were getting ready to discharge Nevaeh and have her pediatrician follow her closely. Distracted by my other cases in the hospital—it had been a very bad week for babies—I agreed with the plan, thinking that with the next admission I would be more aggressive.

Nevaeh was admitted again just a few days later, but this time to die. I was lecturing at grand rounds in the hospital when one of the pediatric residents told me Nevaeh was back and not expected to live. I will never forget the visceral pain I felt, the disorientation, the guilt, both then and even now.

I met with Nevaeh's mother again. She told me that Nevaeh had been lying on the bed acting fine. Suddenly, she choked and turned blue. But this time, she did not come quickly back around as she had always done in the past. When the ambulance arrived, Nevaeh had no heartbeat and was not breathing. The paramedics were able to restart her heart, but she never woke.

Her final hours of life took on an all-too-familiar inevitability. In less than a day, her weakly beating heart finally caught up with her already dead brain.

All the investigations after that—the case reviews, the autopsy, the police—were thorough yet futile. Even though we all believed that this mother had killed her baby, we could not prove it.

During my almost unendurable agony at what had happened, my sleepless ruminations about what I might have done differently, I visited her grave. I have never been to a baby's grave before or since. It was so small, almost invisible amid the multitude of adult graves. There should never be a baby grave. I will never forget that grave. I will never forget Nevaeh.


Munchausen syndrome by proxy is one of the most difficult diagnoses for a child abuse pediatrician to make. Because these parents are so skilled at impostering mothering, in a sort of "perversion of good mothering" (Schreier 1992), as psychiatrist Herb Schreier has eloquently put it, because, even when we are most skeptical, we still remain at heart dangerously gullible, the diagnosis is often missed entirely. Proof is often elusive. Even when found, for example, in a blood urine test, such proof is sometimes dismissed by the very doctors who ordered the test. Because the parent looks so good, "saint-like," the assumption is that the test is wrong.

Baron Munchausen was an 18th-century German nobleman who told many outrageous and seemingly impossible stories about himself. He was a superb liar. In 1951, Richard Asher published a paper in *The Lancet* titled "Munchausen's Syndrome." The opening paragraph is worth quoting in part. "Here is described a common syndrome. Like the famous Baron von Munchausen, the persons affected have always travelled widely; and their stories, like those attributed to him, are both dramatic and untruthful. Accordingly the syndrome is respectfully dedicated to the baron, and named after him."

Asher's fantastic liars fooled medical providers into performing multiple unnecessary tests and procedures on them often, it seemed, to gain sympathetic medical attention.

In 1977, Roy Meadow published a paper also in *The Lancet*, titled "Munchausen Syndrome by Proxy: The Hinterland of Child Abuse" (Meadow 1977). His opening paragraph is also worth repeating: "A case is reported in which over a period of six years, the parents systematically provided fictitious information about the child's symptoms and tampered with the urine specimens to produce false results. This caused the girl innumerable investigations and anesthetic, surgical, and radiological procedures. This long-running saga of hospital care was reminiscent of the Munchausen Syndrome, in this case by proxy."

In a classic 1987 literature review of Munchausen syndrome by proxy, Donna Rosenberg from the University of Colorado Health Science Center wrote about what she termed a "Web of Deceit" (Rosenberg 1987). She described a syndrome that was characterized by illness in a child which is faked and/or produced by a caretaker and presentation of the child for medical care and multiple medical procedures. She also reported that these dramatic symptoms and signs would abate when the child was separated from the perpetrator.

In her review of the published literature, she found 117 children divided almost equally among males and females. Onset of symptoms was usually around one year of age, while diagnosis was often delayed for a year or more. During that time frame, from symptom onset to eventual diagnosis, these children suffered both from unnecessary medical procedures and, in many cases, from direct harm by the parent.

The list of their symptoms these children had included apnea, diarrhea, bleeding, seizures, fever, rash, stupor, and vomiting. Some of the methods that were used to produce these symptoms included poisoning with a blood thinner, poisoning with a laxative or emetic, and suffocation. In some cases, the perpetrator was found to have made up the illness. The harm to these children came from multiple unnecessary medical procedures.

Of the 117 children, 10 died, while at least 8 percent of survivors had significant long-term health problems. Perpetrators were always mothers, in most cases biological mothers, in a few adoptive mothers. Recently, cases have been reported of males engaging in this form of child abuse. Most mothers were described as affable, friendly, and socially adept. Criminal conviction occurred in only 8 percent of cases.

Over the years, the name of this disorder would change from Munchausen syndrome by proxy to pediatric condition falsification to caretaker fabricated illness to, most recently, medical child abuse. But the devastation to the child remains the same, chronic illness, unnecessary medical investigations, psychological trauma, even death.

How can a parent who makes up symptoms harm their child? Consider what happens when a parent tells a medical provider that their child has recurrent vomiting, diarrhea, seizures, or apnea, even though they don't. The conscientious physician would be remiss if they did not try to find out what might be causing these symptoms. They would run tests, perform procedures, and, in some cases, operate to diagnose and treat the problem. Thus, a totally well child is hospitalized and, according to Rosenberg, the doctor, "with an eagerness seen as malignant only in retrospect, investigates and reinvestigates, operates, prescribes, and gives attention and solace. The mothers find for themselves a curious sense of purpose and safety in the midst of the disasters which they themselves have created."

Lest there be skepticism about the reality of this form of child abuse, two papers described the results of hospital video surveillance. Roy Meadow (1990) in a paper titled 'Suffocation, Recurrent Apnea, and Sudden Infant Death" describes 27 children who were suffocated by their mothers. The suffocation was established by reliable observation or video recording of suffocation in the hospital, and/or maternal confession. In some cases, Meadow felt that criminal conviction established the fact of suffocation. Even leaving out criminal conviction, 23 of 27 cases had met one or more other diagnostic criteria. Of these 27 children, 9 died. In addition, these 27 children had 18 siblings who died suddenly and unexpectedly.

In a more recent paper, Hall and his colleagues from Children's Healthcare of Atlanta at Scottish Rite and Emery University (Hall et al. 2000) reported on hospital covert video surveillance of suspected cases of Munchausen syndrome by proxy. They found that video surveillance established the diagnosis in several cases. There was video evidence of suffocation in three cases; medication given to the child via mouth or tube in seven cases, and, in one case, the mother was seen injecting her own urine into a child's intravenous line causing infection.

A remarkable article was published in *Pediatrics* in 1997 titled "My Mother Caused My Illness: The Story of a Survivor of Munchausen by Proxy Syndrome" (Bryk and Siegel 1997). In the paper, Mary Bryk courageously told her own story of chronic abuse. Starting at the age of 2 proceeding until the age of 10, she underwent 28 hospitalizations, 24 surgeries, multiple blood transfusions, and several surgical procedures including skin and bone grafts for recurrent infections. What was not known at the time by anyone other than Mary herself was that these injuries and infections were caused by her mother who would use a hammer to create the injuries and a sharp instrument to contaminate the wounds with potting soil and coffee grounds.

---

Munchausen syndrome by proxy can be exceedingly difficult to investigate. Cases are often accompanied by boxes of records with sometimes conflicting information. Record collection and review can take months. Only infrequently can the diagnosis can be definitively established. None of the child abuse doctors I spoke to particularly enjoy this grueling, often unsatisfying, work. Yet, at the same time, they never forget these children.

**Emalee G. Flaherty, MD, Chicago, Illinois**

There's one case that really haunts me. I still wonder what actually happened. The child had a seizure and was found to be hypoglycemic (low blood sugar that caused the seizure). Someone had the presence of mind to draw an extra tube of blood that could be tested later and sent it along with the child to our center. We tested the blood for drugs that might cause a low blood sugar. The tests came back positive, meaning someone had given the child a drug that caused the low blood sugar and the seizure.

We consulted several endocrinologists who agreed the low blood sugar could only have been caused by the child being given a drug. The family denied having anything in their possession that might have done this. Obviously though, someone had given her a drug.

Our child protective service was not used to dealing with this type of problem and, as is often the case, the child was eventually returned home. I wish I knew the final outcome. It still haunts me wondering what had been done to that child and how she eventually turned out. I worry about what's happening to her now, and if she is being protected. Perhaps the poisoning was a one-time thing. Perhaps the drug was mistakenly given to treat an illness. As I think about that child, those are my most optimistic hope.

### Amanda Brownell, MD FAAP, Cincinnati, Ohio

We saw this young boy who we ultimately diagnosed as suffering from medical child abuse. He had a feeding tube, was on oxygen, and was taking multiple medications. In our review, we found no objective evidence that he needed any of these things. There was no evidence he was in pain, no evidence he had a feeding intolerance, and no evidence that he needed oxygen.

His mother had said that he was dying of cancer and receiving end-of-life care. This was patently untrue. She had even posted pictures of him online with his head shaved asking for donations.

One of our biggest concerns during our initial chart review and prior to the hospitalization was the comment about end-of-life care. If the mother was saying her child was dying, even though he was not, what was the end game going to be? Would she cause his death to complete the process?

Children's services were contacted and the child was admitted to the hospital. His mother was not allowed to visit. The change in his condition was immediate and astonishing. He no longer needed oxygen or pain medication. He started eating a normal diet. We had never seen anything so dramatic. It was like night and day.

It was so rewarding to see that, within literally 24 hours, he was now a normal child. Here was a child who had been attached to multiple tubes and lines and not eating, who suddenly was running around the hospital, eating everything he could get his hands on.

I think the social media aspect is fascinating. At what point can we as physicians go online and Google a family or look at their Facebook page or their GoFundMe page? How much does that play into the abuse of the child and help us figure out the parent's motivation?

(Doctor Feldman and colleagues [Brown et al. 2013] recently published a paper titled "Caretaker Blogs in Caregiver Fabricated Illness in a Child: A Window on the Caretaker's Thinking?" The paper reported on three confirmed cases, of what the authors called caretaker fabricated illness, seen at Seattle Children's Hospital. In all three cases, the diagnosis was finally confirmed when the child was separated from the caretaker and recovered from profound illnesses. In all three cases, the mothers described the children as critically ill and nearing death. These blogs on popular social media and fund-raising sites showed a pattern of exaggeration and misrepresentation of the child's symptoms. In some cases, the blogs described frank deception including fabrication of test results. The blogs also revealed an interesting insight into the caretaker. One mother had written about her struggle to have faith in the future recognizing that there would be none for her child.)

**Allison M. Jackson, MD, MPH, Washington, DC**

One case I had was that of a seven-year-old little boy. A psychologist called me concerned about Munchausen by proxy because the guardian said he had all these behavioral problems, none of which the psychologist saw. The child had been given a host of diagnoses including seizure disorder, asthma, reflux, agoraphobia, autism, and ADHD (attention deficit hyperactivity disorder) and he was on an ungodly number of medications.

I told the psychologist that, if he had suspicion, it was like any other form of child abuse, and he had to report it to CPS. At the same time, we talked about how complicated these cases can be and how child protective services do not always know what to do with them.

I called the hotline CPS supervisor myself, alerting her to the incoming call from the psychologist. I wanted to make sure they would take his call seriously and not just dismiss it because they didn't know what to do with it.

Ultimately, the plan was to hospitalize him so that all of the necessary subspecialists could make their recommendations about the safest way to discontinue his medications if they weren't necessary. Shortly after he was hospitalized, he was off all medications. He had no behavioral symptoms. He was acting like a normal child.

When I reviewed all of his medical records, I was shocked. His illnesses started in infancy with apnea and feeding problems, a pattern of symptoms so typical of medical child abuse.

I remember going to visit him in his room. His bed was filled with toys. Everybody in the hospital was showering him with way more gifts than he needed. A couple of things really struck me when I saw him. He had not been to school, because his mother kept making all these excuses about why he couldn't go. He had been basically living in his bedroom at home or in a hospital bed.

When I saw him, he was playing a handheld videogame. I looked at it and noticed that it was in French. I could tell that the language did not matter since he could not read. I asked him if he had any books to read at home. He said, "Yes." I asked him how many and he said, "One." I asked him what book and he said, "The Cat in the Hat." I love the *Cat in the Hat*, too, but I'm thinking a seven-year-old should be past that, at least I would hope they would be.

He was adopted by a relative and no longer had any unsupervised contact with his mother. He did really well. By the end of the school year, he was reading *Harry Potter*.

### Christine Barron, MD, Providence, Rhode Island

In one of our cases, a child came into the hospital with an infection. But, while we gathered the family medical history, her mother reported that all of the children in the home had something medically wrong with them. This raised my concern. While we were treating this first child for her infection, her sibling came into the hospital with, according to mom, a "kidney infection." The mother said this second child's doctor had sent her to the hospital, but, when we talked to that doctor, he denied even seeing the child much less sending her to the hospital. We admitted her anyway as a "social admission," so we would be able to observe her and gather data. It was just too concerning.

This second child was so cute. She kept saying her "skinnys" hurt. That's what she called her kidneys, her "skinnys."

Later, her mother was overheard in the bathroom saying to her, "Take this." The child was heard replying, "I don't want it." I was called by nursing and immediately went to their hospital room. When they came out of the bathroom, we spoke with the mother who said she was just giving her daughter a vitamin pill. We reminded the mother that hospital rules forbid any outside medications, even vitamins.

The following day, the same thing happened again in the bathroom. The mother was overheard telling her daughter to "take this." I went into the room and asked the mother if she had given her daughter anything in the bathroom. She nervously said no and rushed out of the hospital. The child said to me, "I don't feel well" and promptly vomited. Since this child had no identified medical problems and no reason to feel sick or vomit, I grabbed a basin. She vomited again, this time into the basin.

One minute the child was fine and then all of a sudden she is vomiting. I suspected her mother had given her ipecac (medication once used to induce vomiting if someone took too many pills). I spoke to our toxicologist and she helped me figure out how to test the vomit. The testing had to be done at an outside lab. They would only test the specimen if we provided payment up front. I gave them my credit card even though I did not know how much they were going to charge. They charged $1,000 to the card then they ran the test. As I suspected, the vomit contained ipecac. The hospital did reimburse me.

After obtaining this information, I met with the mother. She said she had gotten the ipecac online to take as a diet supplement for herself. She would not admit to giving ipecac to her child but we had enough information to place all her children into protective custody for safety.

I saw a baby once who the mother said was having seizures. She described in textbook detail the infant's seizures. The infant was started on Keppra (an anti-seizure medication) by neurology, despite a normal EEG. Because no one else had witnessed the seizures and because of the normal brain wave study, we took her off the Keppra in the hospital. We put a full-time sitter with her so that we could see what mom was talking about if she had a seizure.

Nothing happened. The mother then said maybe it wasn't seizures but a behavioral reaction to reflux known as Sandifer syndrome. The neurologist thought that was reasonable and was ready to discharge the child with the mother. I convinced him not to do that. This mother was not describing a behavioral reaction to reflux. She was describing textbook seizures.

The child was placed with an aunt and did quite well. Her mother went into therapy and eventually admitted to making up the seizures. She said she had been so afraid that something was wrong with her child that she just wanted someone to listen to her and take her seriously.

The baby has now been reunited with her mother and has done great. One might argue that she remains at risk. Interestingly, the mother said she would never do such things to her daughter again because "I know they will tell Doctor Barron."

### Kenneth W. Feldman, MD, Seattle, Washington

Medical child abuse (MCA) has been considered an infrequent problem. More recently, we are seeing children with MCA who do not have parent-induced illness, but instead have either falsification of history or exaggeration of a real illness. However, all forms of illness falsification or fabrication drive excess medical investigation and treatment. Our complex medical systems with multiple specialists, who cross-refer patients without going through the primary care provider, seems particularly vulnerable to this type of parent behavior. We've had a number of children who have central lines, chronic narcotic treatment, are completely bedridden, and unable to take anything by mouth. A week after their mother had been excluded from the hospital, they were not only weaned from all drugs, but were running down the halls eating whatever they could get their hands on. Once the situation is recognized and the child is allowed to be him or herself, it's like watching Lazarus rising from the dead.

We've had a few outright confessions, but it's rare. We have also had a few deaths, including one when a parent pushed a syringe of air through the central line and caused an air embolism.

We published a case report in 1988 about an infant who had been repeatedly poisoned with ipecac. This child was the last of six children to be serially abused. One of the children had been chronically poisoned with phenobarbital (a drug used to treat seizures), while three had experienced diarrhea and failure to thrive induced by secret administration of laxatives (Feldman, Christopher, and Opheim 1989).

(Doctor Feldman's chilling case report published in 1989 noted that an infant girl had been hospitalized multiple times for unexplained vomiting and failure to thrive [failure to gain weight]. There was a suspicion of ipecac poisoning because her older siblings had been poisoned. However, all the tests of her urine were negative. Months later, a sample of her vomit was tested and ipecac was found. The child was removed from her mother. She stopped vomiting and grew. Her mother received therapy for bulimia. At the time of the report, this child had been returned home after six months in foster care. Buried in the report is a description of her younger brother having frequent vomiting and apneic spells. These spells only occurred when the baby was alone with his mother. There were concerns that the mother was inducing the apnea in the infant but no proof was found.)

## About Lee

I saw my first case of Munchausen syndrome by proxy in 1975, three years before Meadow's paper during my pediatric residency. Unfortunately, neither I nor anyone else who cared for this critically ill seven-month-old infant had the slightest suspicion. She kept returning to the hospital with unexplained bouts of diarrhea and weight loss. We feared for her life, particularly since her sibling had died at the age of three of the same mysterious illness.

I remember sitting at her bedside with her mother in the intensive care unit. My memory of her mother was that she was a saint, attending to every need of her ill child. No test we ordered, and we ordered many, helped us. No procedure we performed, and we performed many, helped her. We would hydrate her and feed her. She would improve enough to go home only to return several days later sicker than ever. Eventually, she did not return to our hospital, and I moved on to other cases.

In 1977, the year Meadow's paper was published, another little-noticed paper appeared in a medical journal describing an infant who'd been hospitalized with unexplained diarrhea (Fleisher and Ament 1977). I am not sure what drew me to this particular paper, but as I read it, I realized that this was the very infant girl whose bedside I had sat at for so many nights.

The paper told a chilling story. Several months after I took care of her, this infant ended up at a specialty gastroenterology service in another city. This was the third major medical center evaluation for this nearly one-year-old infant. An attentive medical student noticed that her diaper was sometimes turning red. Phenolphthalein (a common laxative and a red dye under certain acidic conditions such as mixed with urine) was found when her diaper was tested. There was no reason for an infant with intractable diarrhea to have a laxative in her system. It could only have come from someone administering it to her.

Her mother was no longer allowed to visit unsupervised and the child quickly recovered. She fully recovered later in the care of her father. Her mother did admit to poisoning her with Ex-Lax. It turned out that her mother had been trying to kill her with a common over-the-counter laxative just as she had likely killed her brother.

I've seen several cases since that time including a mother who serially poisoned her daughters from early infancy to toddlerhood with ipecac, causing vomiting and failure to thrive. Once the next infant came along, the poisoning switched to that infant. The diagnosis was ultimately made when the fourth child developed not only vomiting and failure to thrive but a cardiomyopathy. Her attending gastroenterologist had come from a center where several such cases had been identified as caused by ipecac. When we tested her urine, we indeed found ipecac. Even more bizarre cases have been reported in the medical literature. But for me the strangest, most frightening, and ultimately most satisfying case was Lee.

When I first met Lee, he was a critically ill 14-year-old boy. He'd been diagnosed with a rare mitochondrial disorder and was expected to soon die. He had become unexpectedly lethargic, almost comatose during the current hospitalization. This was the second time this had happened. A few weeks earlier, his mother had, perhaps inadvertently, caused his symptoms by giving him morphine and Valium, presumably to make him comfortable. She was told to stop giving these drugs to him. She agreed.

Now he was back with the same symptoms. His mother denied giving him drugs yet morphine and Valium were found in his urine. This aroused the suspicion of the intensive care doctor who called me. His suspicion fell short of thinking the mother had caused the original illness, but as I heard the story I wondered how far down the rabbit hole this case might take me.

I called child protective services and the police before even meeting with the mother. I wanted to have them present if my suspicions were correct. I would not make the same mistake I made with Nevaeh.

When I got to the hospital, I met Lee's mother. We talked for a long time about Lee and about his brother Billy, who, she told me, had died from a similar mysterious illness years earlier. Lee's mother seemed very concerned and caring, eager to take care of her dying son. She was suspicious of my questions. Strikingly, she told me that she had been through such an investigation twice before, once with Billy, and again when Lee was a baby. She said that she had been cleared by the doctors and by psychologists both times of what she was told was an evaluation for Munchausen syndrome by proxy.

She said that after Billy was born, he started having spells where he stopped breathing and turned blue. Despite multiple hospitalizations no cause was ever found. After a while the breathing problems stopped, but then severe diarrhea started. By the time he was a year old, he stopped growing. When he was three years old, his mother took him to one of the leading pediatric hospitals in the country. During this hospitalization, one of many, someone thought to test his urine for phenolphthalein (a common over-the-counter laxative). Surprising all his doctors, the test came back positive. But, because Billy's mother was so convincing in her concern for Billy, his doctors chose to ignore the results. They concluded that the test result must have been a lab error. Another test done several days later was negative for phenolphthalein, but by then Billy's mother had long known about the results of the first test.

Mental health providers and even a child abuse doctor wrote in Billy's hospital chart that this could not possibly be Munchausen by proxy because Billy's mother presented so well, so caring, and "saint-like." Billy continued to fail despite everything his doctors tried. Finally, out of desperation, the doctors asked Billy's mother to leave the hospital "for a few days." Billy died a short while later. An autopsy was done but nothing was found. Astonishingly, no drugs or toxins were tested for, not even phenolphthalein.

I learned some of this from Lee's mother. I learned much more when, buried in the three-foot stack of medical records I later reviewed, I came upon a journal article about Billy and Lee, pseudonyms assigned to these children by the authors of the paper. The paper was titled "A 3-year-old boy's chronic diarrhea and unexplained death" (Sugar et al. 1991). The story was riveting and horrifying. The paper noted that Munchausen by proxy could well have been the cause of Billy's death. In the last sentence of the paper, the authors asked one final unanswered question, "What about Lee?" What indeed?

Lee started having apnea spells in infancy. He saw multiple specialists in multiple centers. Later Lee, like his brother, developed diarrhea and stopped growing. Somewhere along the way, Lee was given a tentative diagnosis of a mitochondrial disorder, but the diagnosis was never clearly proven.

Now Lee, a 14-year-old, tube fed for a year and bedridden for two, was in my hospital waiting to die. His mother had just purchased a cemetery plot for him. She had written an essay on what it felt like to be the caretaker of a dying child. She used a lovely metaphor of being on a trip to a foreign country, but not the one she had expected to go to. She wrote in clear and simple prose how lonely and disorienting it was to be in the wrong country, yet in some ways how beautiful. She said that she could not mourn the fact she had gone to a different country, because then she would never be able to enjoy the very lovely, very special things about this new, unplanned country. It was almost like she was describing being Alice in Wonderland.

Down the rabbit hole indeed! Only this time, we were going with her.

There was only one thing to do. I told Lee's mother she had to leave the hospital. The detective and I escorted her back to Lee's room where she said goodbye and left. As she left, the detective asked if he could search her purse. She refused.

Within three days of his mother's leaving, Lee, bedridden for two years, got up from bed. Within a week, having been tube fed for a year, he was running around the hospital eating peanut butter and jelly sandwiches. He was never sick again.

What had caused Lee's illness that looked so much like a metabolic disorder but wasn't? Besides the morphine and Valium, we also found aspirin in his blood. In sufficient quantities, aspirin could easily mimic a metabolic disorder. Lee's mother had first chronically poisoned him with aspirin. Then she tried to kill him with morphine and Valium. Her parental rights were ultimately terminated, but she was never prosecuted. No jury would believe a mother could do this to her son.

Some years later, I attended a lecture by Herb Schreier from Children's Hospital Oakland on Munchausen syndrome. I was stunned to hear him talk about a child who had to be Lee. After the lecture, we talked and both of us realized that indeed he had been briefly and informally consulted when Lee was two years old. We agreed to write the case up as a letter to the editor of the *Journal of the American Academy of Child and Adolescent Psychiatry*, the very journal that had published the original case description (Schreier and Ricci 2002). We wrote the letter to alert them to what had happened over the ensuing years with Lee. We also wanted to inform readers of some of the problems in the original evaluations of Billy and Lee, that a psychological evaluation of a mother can never be used to eliminate the possibility of Munchausen, that the toxicology evaluation of Billy was woefully inadequate, that a mother's behavior and appearance such as loving and attentive should never be interpreted to mean that Munchausen is impossible.

Several years later, I received a letter from Lee asking if I would support his entry into the military. I replied that I would. I wanted to ask him how he was doing. Even more, I wanted to ask him how he felt about what had been done to him. I never heard back.

Parenting exists along a continuum with appropriately responsive parents in the middle. On one side of this middle lies lackadaisical or sometimes inattentive, but still adequate parenting, on the other side lies overattentive, overanxious, even unconsciously exaggerating, but still adequate parenting. The extremes at either end of the line, however, contain something entirely different. Beyond overattentive, overanxious, and exaggerating lies the topic of this chapter, a parent who intentionally fabricates or induces illness in his or her child. Beyond lackadaisical or inattentive lies the grossly neglectful parent and the horribly neglected child. Serious neglect remains by far the most prevalent form of child abuse and in many ways the most devastating.

## CHAPTER FOUR

# The Hidden Ravages of Neglect

There are many definitions of child neglect, some more accurate than others. Google would define child neglect as the failure of caretakers to provide adequate emotional and physical care for a child. This is adequate as far as it goes but, as with many things medical, Doctor Google leaves much unanswered.

Federal statutes (Child Welfare Information Gateway 2013, 2016) define neglect as the failure of a parent or other person with responsibility for the child to provide needed food, clothing, shelter, medical care, or supervision *to the degree that the child's health, safety, and well-being are threatened with harm* [emphasis added]. This definition describes an essential component of neglect, the effect on the child.

An even better definition is that of the National Child Abuse and Neglect Data Set (NCANDS) (U.S. Department of Health and Human Services, Administration for Children and Families, Administration on Children, Youth and Families, Children's Bureau 2016). NCANDS defines neglect as the failure of the caretaker to provide needed care, although financially able to do so. Neglect is also usually typified by *an ongoing pattern* [emphasis added]. Categories include physical, educational, emotional, and medical neglect.

Doctor Howard Dubowitz (Dubowitz et al. 2000) would expand the definition beyond the caretaker by adding that a child's basic needs are not adequately met and *attributable to parent, family or community factors* [emphasis added]. Such basic needs include adequate food, health care, clothing, nurturance, protection, supervision, education, and a home. He also adds that such omissions must result in actual or potential harm to the child.

Three million children, 4 percent of all children in the United States, are abused or are at significant risk of abuse every year (Sedlak et al. 2010). Of these, more than 60 percent are victims of neglect.

Neglect can reveal itself in a multitude of ways: lack of cognitive development, lack of medical care, poor speech, poor dental care, and, in its most visible form, as devastating failure to thrive (failure to grow). The long-term ravages of neglect are far worse than for any other form of child abuse and include poor physical growth, impaired cognitive development, and impaired behavioral development. Yet, neglect is often invisible, even to many professionals.

When lecturing pediatric residents, I ask them how many of the following cases, taken from one month of child abuse reports from my institution, involve neglect:

- Two siblings, age seven months and two years, suffer from severe nutritional and developmental failure to thrive.
- The mother of a physically abused three-year-old leaves the emergency room to "shoot up" Ritalin (a stimulant) while her child is being diagnosed and treated.
- A two-year-old is in the intensive care unit after ingesting clonidine (a sedative). This was the child's second ingestion.
- A two-month-old is critically ill in the hospital with a respirator infection. The parents never visit.
- A pregnant woman is admitted to the hospital with a street drug overdose.
- A baby is born drug affected after the mother used illegally purchased oxycodone.
- A baby is born drug affected. Her mother who takes prescribed methadone had received no prenatal care.

Of course, the answer I am looking for is all of them.

I also describe for them the story of a four-year-old now in state custody. The family of this child had been known to the state child welfare system for many years. The parents had already lost four other children to state custody. After the birth of this child, the state became involved with the family, yet again, because of neglect concerns. The parents were reported to smoke marijuana daily and often drank to intoxication. They were seen leaving the child alone for hours at a time. They had been offered multiple services including child development, family preservation, visiting nurse, and parenting education. The services were usually refused. Even when services were accepted, providers found the parents difficult, if not impossible, to work with. Several referrals had been made to child development services, yet the family never followed through.

Even a hard-to-get referral to a developmental pediatrician had been offered and the family failed three times to show up for the appointment. These parents, despite a long history of child protective service involvement and despite the multitude of involved professionals who tried to work with them, never acknowledged that there were any problems in their home.

Finally, in state custody at age four, this child received a comprehensive psychological and medical assessment. She is profoundly developmentally delayed, inadequately immunized, and has rotting teeth. She barely speaks and barely walks. The immunizations and the teeth are easy fixes. The developmental delays are more challenging. In my most cynical mood, I might say she is doomed to a life of learning difficulties, behavioral problems, perhaps criminality, and substance abuse. Should she have children of her own, they likely await a similar fate. How could this have happened? How could this have gone on so long?

Neglect is rarely seen for what it is. Usually, it is something else that brings the plight of the children to the attention of providers, for example, exposure to a sex offender, an injury, or nutritional failure to thrive. Twenty years ago, Doctor Charles Johnson, a colleague of mine, penned a cartoon showing an abused child in a hallway surrounded by closed doors. In the first frame, the child said he had been neglected. No door opened. In the second frame, the child said he had witnessed domestic violence. No door opened. In the third frame, the child said he had been exposed to drug abuse. No door opened. Finally, in the last frame, the child, now with a light bulb over his head, said he had been sexually abused. Every door burst open and outpoured provider after provider.

I was struck by this cartoon then and I am struck by it now. It seems that we providers can only think concretely. Neglect is too nebulous, too vague, for us to grasp. And so the doors stay closed until by lucky or unlucky happenstance something happens that we can understand, like physical or sexual abuse. Howard Dubowitz and others (Dubowitz 2007; Wolock and Horowitz 1984) have used the phrase "the neglect of neglect" to crystalize this issue. A broken bone, bruising, or sexual abuse is concrete and understandable. Neglect is not, and so we, along with everyone else, ignore it until it is often too late.

I am often told by doctors and child welfare professionals alike that a child may have been abused or neglected but that what happened to the child was unintentional. Often abuse and neglect are unintentional, at least in terms of the effects, if not the cause. Surely, it is not the intent of most parents to leave their child developmentally delayed or medically neglected. Nor is it the intent of most parents to cause a broken bone or a serious head injury. But here is the critical point. For the child, intent does not matter. What matters for the child is the effect on them. According to Fong and Christian (2012), a broad view of neglect requires only that a child has unmet basic needs. This view refocuses the attention where it belongs, on the child.

Failure to thrive is the most visible form of the often invisible devastation of neglect: babies with bloated bellies, toothpick limbs, sunken eyes behind blank faces, and apathy, terrible apathy. It is hard to believe this happens in America. Admittedly, not all failure to thrive is that bad, but, even less severe caloric deprivation can have lifelong adverse developmental consequences. Without food, first a baby's body does not grow, then, if food deprivation continues, their brain does not grow.

Broadly speaking, there are two types of nutritional failure to thrive: one organic due to an underlying medical condition like gastrointestinal disease, the other environmental, an otherwise healthy baby simply not being fed enough. There is overlap of course, for example, a child with oral aversion who is also not being fed adequately.

The most common parent and child features of environmental failure to thrive we see in our Failure to Thrive Clinic is an ignoring parent and a nondemanding infant. Often, other social situational risk factors such as domestic violence and substance abuse are present. Occasionally, these infants are also being physical abused. Invariably, they are being developmentally neglected.

Failure to thrive, in its simplest sense, is the failure to gain weight at an acceptable rate. There are more technical definitions involving growth curves and percentiles but in the end all children should follow a standard growth curve that is appropriate to them. Failure to do so for long enough or severe enough is failure to thrive. Risk factors for failure to thrive include poverty, poor bonding, domestic violence, substance abuse, social isolation, mental health problems in the caretaker, disordered feeding techniques, and unusual health and nutrition beliefs.

Failure to thrive is entirely treatable, often without removing a child from their caretakers. All that is required is a caretaker who understands that there is a problem and is willing to engage in services. However, should there be coexistent domestic violence, substance abuse, or physical abuse along with parents who refuse to acknowledge a problem and who refuse to engage in services, then invariably these children need to be placed in a safe, nurturing environment, at least until they have nutritionally recovered. Often this takes many months. In some cases, the risk issues in the birth family are so great, so pervasive, and so untreatable, that children end up permanently removed from their parents.

**Christine Barron, MD, Providence, Rhode Island**

We have seen failure to thrive cases where the parents don't understand the problem because it was never clearly explained to them, or they are not getting the appropriate services to help them fix the problem. In these cases, if the parents work with us, we can correct the failure to thrive and preserve the family. But then there are other cases where the family won't or can't work with us. Even then we try as hard as we can to salvage the family. It doesn't always work.

I had a case of twins who were failing to thrive. It really came down to mom's obsessive compulsive disorder. She just could not stand allowing these toddlers to feed themselves because it would make too much of a mess. Those children eventually went to live with their dad and they grew without any problems.

I had another case of failure to thrive involving twins where the mother said she was feeding them but still they did not grow, even with calorie-boosted formula. Finally, I said to child welfare, "There's no way mom is feeding them what's she saying. It's impossible." When we placed them in care, they grew so incredibly fast that we had to take them off calorie-boosted formula and put them on regular formula. Still they grew and grew and grew. In my report, I wrote, "This proves that if you feed them, they will grow."

**Richard D. Krugman, MD, Aurora, Colorado**

I use this case even now when I give medical students a lecture on abuse. We admitted a three-month-old infant who was still at her birth weight. She was terribly emaciated. Her mother was in her late twenties. There was a two-and-a-half-year-old sibling who we ultimately diagnosed as being emotionally neglected. She would run into anybody's arms just to be with someone, anyone.

I tried to treat the infant outpatient for a few days. She gained a little weight but not enough. So I admitted her to the hospital. In the hospital, she gained two ounces a day, a spectacular amount. Even with that demonstration of the failure of home care, I still thought this child could go home with the parents and be treated by me as an outpatient. We would have a public health nurse to their home two or three times a week. We would have social work and child protective services visit them and I'd see them every week.

I presented this case at our child protective meeting. Doctor Brandt Steele, who was an early pioneering psychiatrist in the field of child abuse at the University of Colorado Hospital Child Protection Team (one of the first three in the United States), was at the conference.

He asked me, "Well, are you sure these are the only two babies that this mother has had?" I said, "I took the history. That's what she said." He said, "Well, I don't believe it. I think she's probably got other children." At that moment, the county child protective worker came into the meeting and told us that she had checked registries in three states. These were not the only two children this mother had given birth to. These were number eight and nine. The first three were abused and taken by child welfare in California. The next two were abused and taken by child welfare in Texas. The next two were born in Kansas, one was removed and one died from what was presumed to be SIDS (sudden infant death syndrome). My two were numbers eight and nine. We later found out that there were contracts for the sale of these two children to a sex ring in Colorado because the parents were running out of money.

I asked Brandt, "How did you know there were other children?" He said, "Well, the fact that this baby is three months old and at birth weight—that suggests to me severe neglect on the part of the mother and therefore a mother who herself had to have been pretty severely abused and neglected. She has no ability to bond with these children. I've never seen a woman who was severely abused as a child who had her first child at the age of 26. She must have started having babies when she was abused as a teenager." Sure enough, she had her first baby when she was 15.

I try to help students understand that the approach to these problems is to understand the history, the complete history. I tell them what Brandt said, "If you don't understand somebody's behavior, you don't have enough history." The only way to get a clear and truthful history in a lot of these cases is to have multiple disciplines assess the family, law enforcement, child protective services, civil and criminal lawyers, psychology, psychiatric, and pediatric medicine.

**Carole Jenny, MD, MBA, Seattle, Washington**

What we're seeing now, which I find terribly discouraging, is healthy adults with unusual nutritional beliefs who feed their infants nutrient poor diets because it is "healthy." We've had two children in the last year who almost died of rickets. They were stunted, couldn't walk or even sit up. Their parents wouldn't feed them anything that wasn't 100 percent pure. They were feeding them some kind of "special milk" that they made themselves that had insufficient calories and no supplemental vitamin D in it. I don't understand it. These were seemingly intelligent parents. One of the mothers was a nurse!

Out here, those who plan to deliver their baby at home often don't give vitamin K at birth. We are seeing vitamin K deficiency brain bleeding. Perfectly lovely little babies are coming in to our hospital at two or three weeks of age devastated from bleeding in their brain. This was 100 percent preventable, if only the babies had been given vitamin K at birth.

**Allison M. Jackson, MD, MPH, Washington, DC**

I saw a school aged child who was referred to me by our emergency room for profound failure to thrive. She had been in the care of her mother who would not let her father visit her. The father went to the school to see her. He found out from the school that she had not been there in months. When the father finally saw his daughter, he was shocked to see how skeletal she looked. He also saw inflicted bruises and scars on her body. He took her to the hospital.

The emergency department called me in a panic. They had never seen a child so emaciated. She was going to be admitted anyway, but I asked if they would send him to my clinic first so I could examine her. I was hoping to avoid meeting directly with the ED staff. They sounded frantic and I knew if I went there I was going to have to debrief with them and I didn't have time to do that. There would be time to talk later about our mutual horror. Now, I just wanted to evaluate her as comprehensively as possible, and document my consultation.

You see those commercials of children in Africa with flies all over them, bloated bellies, stick figure arms and legs, that's what she looked like. Her dad came over with her and looked on in disbelief and guilt. He could not understand what his daughter had experienced to make her look like that, almost dead from starvation.

She had inflicted burns and ligature marks on her wrists and ankles from being bound up. After her admission, when she had gotten some of her strength back, she told me that she had been burned and tied up, beaten, and often left alone all day.

During one of our talks, I asked her if there was anything else I needed to know, if there was anything I had forgotten to ask her. I will never forget her answer. "You're a life-saver," she said. When she said that, I thought to myself, "I think I need to leave the room just for a minute. I'm going to be right back."

Our role is so different from that of other doctors. I'm not an ED (emergency department) doctor. I'm not an ICU (intensive care unit) doctor. I am not in the life-saving business like ED and ICU doctors. But I will never forget what that child said to me about saving her life. That was one of those statements that made me feel good in the midst of all the horror that I see.

She loved her dad, and it was clear her dad loved her, but at that moment he emotionally wasn't in a place to care for her. She ended up going into foster care.

The staff who saw her later in clinic for primary care told me that they had read my note about what she had said to me. They told me, "We were all crying when we read it."

I try to use actual cases to demonstrate teaching points when I teach medical students and other trainees. I think that one of the things we don't do very well as pediatricians is talk to children about their experiences, good and bad. For me, a lesson from this case is to always talk to children. You just want to do right by them. You want to elicit their experiences and paint the picture of their experiences as best as you can and you hope and pray that they can recover from the horror. It was clearly horror for that little girl. She was targeted. It was like in the book *A Child Called It*.

## About Sarah

Sarah, a two-year-old, came into the hospital having failed to thrive almost since birth. She was lethargic, almost catatonic, profoundly delayed, and profoundly underweight, truly skin and bones. She had seemed to grow well on breast milk up to three months of age. Then she stopped growing so that by eight months of age her pediatrician became concerned and suggested supplementing the breast milk with formula. Rather than do that, the family switched doctors.

The second pediatrician, concerned about the weight and about the mother's odd behavior, made a report to child protective services. The family left that practice and went to a third pediatrician. Child protective services opened an investigation but never met the family or even saw the child. They only spoke to the third pediatrician who felt that the child was indeed failing to thrive and that the mother was odd but also felt that he could work with the family. The child was noted to have significant developmental delays, had not been immunized, and had not been receiving vitamin supplement (Vitamin D supplement is essential for babies exclusively breast fed, particularly in states like Maine with limited sunlight in the winter).

The child did grow a bit for a few months but then at 12 months of age, fell like a rock off the growth curve. The family stopped coming to see this third doctor when their daughter was 16 months old. Eventually, five months later, this pediatrician made a report to child protective services.

At 24 months of age, she became acutely ill with a respiratory infection and had to be admitted to the hospital. By the time I saw her, she was suffering from life-threatening failure to thrive, was not ambulatory, and did not speak.

Exclusive breast feeding had likely been responsible for much of her failure to thrive. All the family would have had to do to correct the problem was to supplement the breast feeding with formula. But her mother was absolutely unwilling to accept that there was a problem and was unwilling to engage with any services. She presented in an almost delusional state talking about cereal acting like cement in the baby's stomach. Her thoughts were confused, pressured, and tangential. Often she had to be redirected back to the issue at hand, namely the child's weight and feeding schedule. The baby's father mumbled something about mercury in immunizations, but otherwise seemed uninvolved.

In foster care, Sarah's failure to thrive completely reversed in just a few months. Ultimately, parental rights were terminated and she was adopted.

Why hadn't this family done the right thing? In this case, there was profound mental illness. In others, personality issues prevent the parent from acknowledging a problem and taking appropriate steps to correct it.

Why had it taken so long for the pediatrician to identify this child as critically neglected? I wish I could say this was an unusual case. Many medical providers think that simply by force of will they can influence parental behavior. Sometimes that is true. Often it is not true, and the greater problem is that we rarely recognize our own failure until it is too late.

## About Michael and Bethany

I was asked to see seven-month-old Michael for failure to thrive in the hospital. He had been healthy as a newborn but by two months of age had stopped growing. In the hospital, he gained weight spectacularly.

As I interviewed his parents, I struggled to understand what had happened to Michael. Neither parent drank or did drugs. They had not been previously involved with child welfare or the police. By report there was no domestic violence, but, as is often the case, that may not have been entirely true. Much like child abuse, domestic violence is often hidden behind closed doors inside family homes. In the interview, Michael's father controlled every conversation while his wife sat meekly silent. He was also a harsh disciplinarian of the children.

Neither parent would accept that Michael was underweight, even after I reviewed the stark growth chart with them. They would not accept that anything had to change in their home. They told me that their two-year-old child Bethany was small and that this was normal for their family. I often hear this in cases of failure to thrive and often silently wonder if more than one child suffered from failure to thrive.

So what about Bethany? After looking at her growth chart, I asked that she be admitted to the hospital as well. Her growth chart was worse than her brothers. Her weight had been pretty good up until seven months earlier when her brother was born. Since then however, she had not gained any weight. More striking were her profound delays. Here was a two-year-old who did not talk, walk, or even sit up. She just lay in bed staring at the ceiling, occasionally smiling when spoken to. This was something more than just nutritional failure to thrive. If this was developmental neglect, and later it was clear that it was, this was profound beyond any comparison.

In the hospital, Bethany too spectacularly gained weight and in foster care they both grew like beans. Michael quickly gained developmental milestones. Bethany's developmental recovery has been much slower. Her profound developmental neglect had gone on too long. She may never fully recover.

Even though the children were removed from their parents' care, because of the federal mandate to first pursue reunification, services were put in place to assist the parents in learning how to care for their children. After two years of effort to reunify the children with their parents however, an incident occurred that convinced everyone involved that reunification was not in the best interest of these children.

The children had been returned to the care of their parent for a trial placement. Multiple services were placed in the home and the family was closely monitored. Yet, for an entire day, while their mother was at work, their father tinkered with his car while Michael and Bethany lay unattended in the home. When asked why he did this, he replied that he thought that it was more important to get the car fixed than to care for the children. Even when told this was a serious lapse, he could only stare straight ahead through uncomprehending eyes.

I suppose a psychological evaluation of the father might show why something like this happened. It might show cognitive limitations. It might even show personality issues. Sometimes, though, it is just as important to look on in wonder at the abject inability of some parents to ever get it right. This was one of those times.

Happily both children are now adopted with wonderful parents. One of my great joys in this work is seeing a parent in love with their child, not just loving their child but in love with them. The difference is hard to put into words. Anyone who has witnessed it knows it for what it is, a miracle of profound, selfless attachment. These adoptive parents were in love with these children. It is here that hope for their future rests.

Rarely is failure to thrive intentional, but when it is, it is horrifying to see. In these cases, failure to thrive can turn into psychosocial dwarfism. The child is not just underweight but their linear growth is profoundly stunted as well (Green, Campbell, and David 1984).

## About Damien

Damien weighed 23 pounds when I first saw him in the hospital at age 7. He weighed 23 pounds when he was nine months old. Now, he was 7 years old and he still weighed 23 pounds. He lay quietly in his hospital bed as I entered the room. He looked up and smiled brightly despite looking frail and horribly undernourished. In a chair by his bed sat his "grandmother." The "mother" and "grandmother" appellations are in quotes here because, although they introduced themselves as "mother" and "grandmother," they had no biological or legal relationship to Damien or to his birth mother. They considered themselves caretakers of Damien and his birth mother. No professional ever met Damien's birth mother nor did they even know these adults were not who they said they were, "mother and grandmother."

The consult request came to me despite the fact that this seven-year-old with profound failure to thrive was thought to be suffering from a psychiatric problem causing the failure to thrive. This type of case would normally involve psychiatry and gastroenterology not a child abuse doctor, but there was something odd here that led the hospital doctors to ask me to get involved.

My first impression on entering the hospital room was how tiny Damien was and how out of control his "grandmother" was. The story she told me was of a willfully defiant, almost satanic, child who could vomit on demand, and who never listened, despite being punished by having food withheld. She described him as cunning and manipulative. She alternated between pleading for help and demanding that Damien be discharged, all the while gesticulating wildly. My interview of her was inordinately long and exhausting, but at the end it was clear to me that this child could not be discharged, not until we knew more about this strange family.

Examining Damien confirmed what I had already suspected. His skin literally hung off his bones, his belly was sticking out, and his limbs were thin. There was one other thing, something that I missed on my initial hurried examination under the "grandmother's" watchful eyes. It was something that I only saw when I later reviewed the photographs I had taken. To my horror, there were subtle but definite whipping scars on his buttocks.

The next day I met with Damien's "mother" but, before that, I reviewed his medical records. His primary care doctor had sent him to us because he was at his wits end trying to figure out how to help this presumably profoundly psychiatrically disabled child who could not seem to grow. The records starkly documented that, after nine months of age, Damien stopped gaining weight. At first, he continued to gain in length but after a while that stopped too. He was now only as tall as a three-year-old. His head growth also suffered, though not as bad as it would have had the caloric deprivation started earlier. Most postnatal brain growth occurs in the first 9–12 months of life and then slows thereafter, although brain development, fine and gross motor skills, language, and social skills continue to increase. Even though his head size had not been as profoundly affected as his weight and length, his social and intellectual development was far below normal. He was functioning at the developmental level of a three-year-old.

The records I reviewed revealed a child who had been variously diagnosed by specialists in two major medical centers as having failure to thrive, self-induced vomiting, and severe psychological dysfunction. What stood out for me was how these various specialists arrived at these diagnoses, exclusively from the history given by his fictive relatives. These caretakers were always identified in the records as Damien's mother and grandmother. No one in multiple medical evaluations had discovered that the adults who called themselves Damien's mother and grandmother were neither.

There is an important difference between child abuse pediatrics and traditional medicine. As traditional medical students, we are taught to first take a detailed history, then perform a physical examination guided by the history, and then obtain tests based on the history and physical. At no point in that or subsequent training are physicians taught to question the history. The assumption always is that the patient and the patient's family, in their own self-interest, will tell the truth to the doctor. But what if there is a motivation to lie, to hide or distort information, as, for example, in Munchausen by proxy or in physical abuse?

This is the reason why a carefully constructed lie to a non-forensically trained medical provider usually works. For an experienced forensically trained provider, the only truth is the appearance of the child, what can be seen with the naked eyes. Damien had profound failure to thrive.

Everything else was suspect, including the presumed, but never clinically seen, self-induced vomiting disorder. None of the highly trained, highly skilled providers who had seen Damien over the years ever questioned the truthfulness or accuracy of the history. When faced with a child with obvious profound failure to thrive and a history from his caretakers that the illness was self-induced, questioning the connecting of these dots was understandable and tragically wrong.

Different from "grandmother's" anxious and agitated presentation, Damien's "mother" presented as calm and coherent. When asked specifically about how many children she had and their names, it finally came out that Damien was not the only child in the home. She stated that Damien and his birth mother had been living with her since he was an infant because his birth mother was profoundly limited. She said she had custody of Damien and would bring in the papers to prove it. She never did. As I found out later, such papers did not exist.

The story that eventually emerged, during various child protective and criminal hearings, horrified me, as much by the failure of the child welfare and medical systems that are supposed to protect children as by the horrible starvation and deprivation Damien had experienced.

When Damien was finally allowed to eat, at will in the hospital, he gained six pounds in six days. In foster care after he left the hospital, he gained an additional fourteen pounds in five months. Most surprisingly, given the chronicity of his starvation, he shot up six inches in six months.

Was Damien starved? Was his starvation intentional? Unquestionably, yes and yes. When finally allowed to eat, his failure to thrive disappeared in a matter of months, although his cognitive and developmental deficits never totally resolved. He will require years of developmental and mental health services and, even then, will likely never totally recover.

Why was this done to Damien? Starting at age nine months food was withheld from Damien by these caretakers. Withholding food from Damien was a form of discipline. I am sure to some extent it worked. Children who are not fed become apathetic rather than defiant.

Perhaps Damien was also being kept small to continue his disability checks. Perhaps there was an element of Munchausen by proxy. For myself, I prefer to think of darker forces at work. I believe that what happened to Damien was simply sadistic torture.

This case illustrates intentional starvation, the most extreme form of failure to thrive. It also illustrates how well-meaning and well-trained professionals can miss the obvious. Not only medical professionals but child welfare professionals, who had investigated the home previously, had missed the obvious. Even the court appointed attorney for Damien felt that

Damien must have had had a medical disorder to account for his illness. The only disorder Damien suffered from was intentional starvation.

When I last saw Damien at age 8, his weight was average for his age and his height was much improved, though he was still short. He was actually a bit chunky. He was in school. His attention span had improved. He was in a pre-adoptive placement, and his birth mother was having regular contact with him. She acknowledged that she could not care for him herself due to her own disabilities. She had been just as much a victim as Damien. Both his fictive relatives were charged with assault for starving Damien. Both were convicted and received lengthy prison sentences.

Can families with failure to thrive be treated? Can the family be preserved?

## About Kendra

I was asked to see Kendra, a two-year-old immigrant child, because, as part of the evaluation for failure to thrive at the hospital, x-rays had been obtained that raised a question of fractures. Kendra had grown well until six months of life, but then she plummeted off the curve, so that now at three years her weight was less than it had been at six months. To compound the issue, she continued to be exclusively breast fed with no vitamin supplement. Breast milk is a poor source of vitamin D for babies. So now, not only was she critically underweight, she also had vitamin D deficient rickets. Her x-ray findings were not from abuse but from profound rickets. Somehow this child had not been given routine supplemental vitamin D and had continued to exclusively breast feed, a recipe for disaster since breast milk has little to no vitamin D.

Looking at her, she looked proportionate. She only had not gained weight but, because of the severity of nutritional failure to thrive and the rickets, she had not grown in length. She actually looked like an average six-month-old, except that she was two years old.

The medical staff loathed to call this neglect by the mother; rather they wanted to call it neglect by the medical provider who had let this go on for so long, who had not given the child vitamin D, who had not insisted on milk supplement. True enough. But I was more interested in what the parents would do now to correct the problem.

Things did not go well from there.

Some doctors felt strongly that this was not parental neglect and did not require child protective services involvement. One hospital doctor felt that she knew the mother was not neglectful after she got to know her, this after seeing her maybe 10 minutes a day over a period of one week, and talking with her through an interpreter. The worst part was that I could not get child protective services to understand how ill this child was. The young and inexperienced worker told me that the child looked ok to her, "proportionate." For one of the few times in my career, I honestly did not know what to say to that.

Ultimately, despite my concern and over my objection, the child was discharged to the mother with recommendations for formula supplement and vitamin D replacement. No services were put in the home. The feeling was that this family, once informed of the problem, would do the right thing and follow the medical recommendations. She had gained a pound in just a few days of hospitalization on formula. So, we did know that if she continued to be fed adequately, she should do well at home. I crossed my fingers and hoped for the best.

The best was not to be, not even close. She returned to the hospital two weeks later having lost everything she had gained in the hospital. When carefully questioned, it was clear that her mother did not believe Kendra had ever been underweight. It was clear that she had not followed our nutritional recommendations. I did not believe her when she said the baby was drinking 24 ounces of whole milk a day. Again, despite my strenuous objection, the baby was sent home.

But then, something very surprising and quite wonderful happened. The entire immigrant community took it upon themselves to support and monitor this mother's care of her daughter. Detailed daily food logs were kept by community members. Feedings were supervised. The baby grew. In four months, she gained eight pounds and her rickets resolved. Best of all, and despite my initial serious misgivings, she was able to stay with her family.

In this case, the community rallied around this baby and family. Sometimes it indeed takes a village. I wish I could say this always works but it is entirely dependent on the willingness of families to accept services and the willingness and availability of the village of professionals and nonprofessionals to help.

Neglect, failure to thrive, even sexual and physical abuse are treatable. Death is not. It is the end of everything. It cannot be reversed, only mourned and remembered. Perhaps, if the lessons of the death are learned and taken to heart, future children can be saved from the same fate. At least that is the hope.

## CHAPTER FIVE

# Child Abuse Fatalities: The Anatomy of Death

A child's death from abuse or neglect can take many forms. In 1988, Doctor Richard Krugman from the C. Henry Kempe National Center for the Prevention and Treatment of Child Abuse and Neglect published a paper on fatal child abuse (Krugman 1988). The paper offered a detailed analysis of 24 deaths over a two-year period. Krugman noted that, in many of these cases, the predisposing child factor for infants less than 12 months was inconsolable crying, while for those over 12 months it was a toileting accident. Head injury accounted for 17 of the 24 deaths. Thirteen children lived with married parents and in six of these cases, the perpetrator was the father. Eleven children lived with their unmarried mother and in seven of these homes the children were killed by a boyfriend.

I have often remarked that no one kills a sleeping baby. This is not in any way to blame the baby. Invariably though, there is some tension between a caretaker and a child that leads a caretaker to maim, if not kill an infant.

In a paper on risk factors, Schnitzer and Ewigman identified 149 inflicted injury deaths over eight years in Missouri (Schnitzer and Ewigman 2005). The majority of known perpetrators were the child's father or the mother's boyfriend. Children living with an unrelated male in the home were 50 times more likely to die of inflicted injuries than children residing with two biological parents. Children in a home with a single parent and no other adults were at no increased risk of death.

The publication "We Can Do Better: Child Abuse and Neglect Deaths in America" reported that, in 2008, 1,740 children died from abuse in the

United States (Every Child Matters Education Fund 2010). In that year, the child abuse fatality rate in the United States was 2.4 per 100,000 children, 3 times higher than Canada's and 11 times higher than Italy's. The United States ranked first in comparison to other resource-rich democracies in the rate of child abuse deaths. The authors felt this disparity was because, different from the United States, other democracies have social policies in support of families such as child care, universal health insurance, paid parental leave, and visiting nurses.

According to the report of the 2016 Commission to Eliminate Child Abuse and Neglect Fatalities, four to eight children die every day from abuse and neglect in the United States (Commission to Eliminate Child Abuse and Neglect Fatalities 2016). Half of these children have not yet reached, nor will they ever reach, their first birthday.

This commission also found that a call, any call, to a child protective hotline is the best predictor of a child's potential risk of death from an injury before age five. It does not matter whether the call is substantiated for abuse or even assigned for investigation. It mattered only that someone, anyone picked up the phone and called child protective services about a child.

Although many children who die from abuse and neglect are already known to child protective services, some are not. However, most of these latter children are known to other professionals such as health-care providers. This highlights the importance of coordinated and multisystem efforts, something that is sorely lacking in our child welfare system, the commission felt. Also, according to the commission, 70 percent of child maltreatment fatalities involve neglect. Many of these deaths occur in families challenged by the stresses of poverty.

Finally, the commission report noted that, even though we know quite a bit about what puts a child at risk for death, we know very little about preventing it. The authors do cite the Nurse-Family Partnership, an intensive program of nurse home visitors, as an evidence-based practice shown to reduce fatalities (Donelan-McCall, Eckenrode, and Olds 2009).

A recent paper looked at the relationship between poverty level (based on federally defined poverty thresholds) by county and child abuse fatality rates in the same counties (Farrell et al. 2017). The authors found that during the study years of 1999 to 2014, 11,000 children died from abuse in the United States, for an overall rate of 3.5 per 100,000 children 0–4 years of age. Counties with the greatest amount of poverty had greater than three times the fatality rate (4.5/100,000) than counties with the lowest poverty concentration (1.3/100,000). The paper notes that the association of community poverty with child abuse fatalities could be in part caused by the lack of available community resources coupled with significant environmental risk factors.

The most common cause of inflicted death in babies is head trauma. Attempts at preventing abusive head trauma through parent education were at first encouraging but most recently disappointing. Starting in the early 1990s, attempts were made to inform parents of the dangers of shaking an infant in the hopes that such information would have an impact on the devastating consequences of shaking an infant (Showers 1992) In 2005, Mark Dias and colleagues published the results of a prevention program implemented in upstate New York (Dias et al. 2005). After the birth of their baby, parents were shown a video about the adverse effects of shaking. They were also asked to sign a document stating they would not shake their baby. During the 5 years of the program, over 60,000 parents were educated in an 8 county region of western New York State. The authors reported that, following the program, the annual incidence of abusive head trauma decreased by 47 percent. This was an astounding result for an education program. On the heels of this study, multiple programs were implemented throughout the country, including one called "The Period of PURPLE Crying" from the National Center on Shaken Baby Syndrome (Barr et al. 2009).

Maine implemented this program several years ago with some fanfare and high hopes. But the numbers did not drop in Maine, nor did they drop in subsequent studies elsewhere including a recent study in Pennsylvania that educated over one million parents. The authors, including the very same Doctor Dias who had published the earlier New York study, found no difference in the incidence of abusive head trauma hospitalizations between families who got the information and those who did not (Dias et al. 2017). In an accompanying editorial, Doctor John Leventhal of Yale suggested that after birth education may not be enough (Leventhal 2017). He offered some suggestions. Education must come from multiple sources: hospitals, doctors' offices, family members, and the media, for example. It may also not be enough to just tell parents to not shake their babies when they are frustrated. One of the problems is that shaking works. It stuns the baby's brain so that they stop crying. An alternative approach might be to teach parents how to manage their feelings of frustration using such techniques as reflective parenting. Paid parental leave, as demonstrated in California, may be associated with a reduction in the rates of abusive head trauma (Klevens et al. 2016). Home visitation programs that support parents might be helpful. Finally, Leventhal suggests that educational programs aimed at preventing abusive head trauma must focus on the most likely perpetrator, the male in the home.

In the meantime, while prevention strategies continue to evolve and while comprehensive prevention remains frustratingly just outside our grasp, it is equally important that we not forget, indeed that we bear witness to, children who have died, and to those families irreparably damaged by that loss.

---

**Christine Barron, MD, Providence, Rhode Island**

I saw a very young infant who died of abusive head trauma. She had so many injuries. Worst of all, she had healing adult bite marks on her body. When I looked at her records, it turned out that she had been seen by another hospital for these same bite marks. They had documented injuries but they did not know they were bite marks so they sent her for blood tests thinking maybe she had a bleeding disorder. The injuries were clearly adult bite marks. They missed the diagnosis.

When I talked to the baby's mother who had witnessed the bites, she said to me, "Well, the other hospital didn't pick that up."

I said, "Well you didn't tell them the truth."

She said to me, "But if I did, you would have placed my baby in custody."

I replied, "If I did, your baby would be alive."

I was really frustrated. That was a terrible case. To me the most frustrating part of my work is when obvious inflicted injuries are missed, misdiagnosed, or simply dismissed by medical professionals and then the baby comes back with further serious injury or death. There are unfortunately too many of those kinds of cases. If a child abuse pediatrician had seen this child with the bite marks while she was still alive, she would not have died.

People say to me, "Well, don't you train everyone?" I tell them, "Oh my goodness. Do you know how much training we do? We do training upon training upon training."

I can't tell you how many times I hear, "But this is a nice family." My response is always, "I don't care. Nice has nothing to do with it." I will argue that I don't care where the family is from, either. I don't care if they're from South Providence or if they're from Barrington. To me, every case should be treated the same.

I approach all cases the same, I collect all of the clinical puzzle pieces, the nature of the injuries, the likely mechanism of the injuries, the developmental ability of the child, all of the medical information. I work with a multidisciplinary team and identify a list of all possible diagnosis before I make my diagnosis.

**Richard D. Krugman, MD, Aurora, Colorado**

I was brought a case by a Colorado Springs attorney who said to me, "I think the DA (District Attorney) has got the wrong person. I've read a lot about child abuse and my client is this wonderful woman who was babysitting for this young boy. She's married, has a three-year-old girl and they're upper middle class. The child's mother is an African-American, in the military, under a lot of stress, and she was abused herself as a child. I just don't believe that the babysitter harmed this child. I think the mother did it the night before and the baby just died at the babysitter's."

On reviewing the records it was clear to me that the mother was stressed. She was about to be deployed and because she was going to a war zone she could not take her baby with her. She was going to have to leave her son with her own parents who had not been the best parents for her.

It was also clear that the boy was fine when dropped off at the sitters. He could not have already sustained an ultimately fatal abdominal injury. The babysitter agreed that he was fine when he was dropped off. While he was at the sitters he had breakfast, played for a while, then he took a nap. When he woke up from his nap, he had a bowel movement in his diaper. The sitter took him to the bathroom and changed him. Then she put him in the tub. She said he slipped and hit his head on the bathtub but seemed okay. She put him in a high chair and gave him a snack. About a half hour later, he slumped over unconscious. She called 911 and the ambulance took him to the base hospital. He had swelling on the left side of his head where she said his head had hit against the bathtub.

They didn't have a CT (Computerized Tomography, an x-ray technique used in this case to examine the skull and brain) scanner at the base hospital so they transferred him to a hospital that did. The CT there showed a skull fracture and a small subdural hematoma. In the ambulance on the way back to the base hospital, he had a cardiac arrest and died. They had all missed the ruptured liver, spleen and mesenteric artery. He basically bled into his abdomen in the ambulance and died.

After I read the case, I said to the lawyer, "The babysitter had to have done it. A child couldn't have these severe abdominal injuries, then eat breakfast, and play. Something happened in the bathroom."

He went back to his client and spoke with her. She ultimately confessed to what she had done. She told the police that, after she changed the boy's diaper, he pooped again. She became irritated because her three-year-old was fussing in another room. As she spoke to the boy, he looked at her with a funny smile. A psychiatrist who evaluated her prior to sentencing asked her, "What do you mean, a funny smile?" She said, "It was a smile like my uncle had." It turned out her uncle had sexually abused her and he always had this smile on his face while he abused her. She had never told anyone about this. In that moment, she saw her uncle in this little boy. She lifted him up, smashed his head against the bathtub, and then stomped on his abdomen. Then she sort of came around, cleaned him up, and put him in the high chair. A short time later he slumped over.

I present this case to students as if they were a mock jury. I give them the case details and ask them, "How many of you think the mother did it?" The mother's African-American, 19, abused as a child, and stressed. About a third of the class raises their hands and thinks that the mother did it. A third thinks the babysitter did it. A third do not raise their hands at all, they have no idea. Then I ask them, "What else do you want to know?"

### Alex V. Levin, MD, MHSc, Philadelphia, Pennsylvania

I interviewed a mom when I was in my first year as a child abuse pediatrician. Her child was lying dead in the emergency room. I took her to my office to talk and I asked her what happened. She looked at me with a blank, emotionless expression on her face and said, "I shook him and I shook him and I shook him until he was no more"

I can see her now, in my mind's eye, right now, I can see that moment. I could draw you a picture of it.

How horrible. The honesty, the brutal honesty, the rawness stuck me. My first thought though was not, "You evil person". My first thought was overwhelming sadness for what this person had become. Who was she? How did she get to this point? I'm sure she wasn't born a murderer. That's where I really crystallized the idea that this isn't about bad people doing bad things.

### Desmond K. Runyan, MD, DrPH, Denver, Colorado

I've often talked with my social work and legal colleagues about a particular problem in abusive head trauma criminal prosecution. A father is convicted and goes to jail. But then not only does he suffer but the mother suffers as well. She has, in all likelihood, a handicapped child. She's impoverished. She may have lost health insurance. She has no income because the father was the only one who worked. Even if she worked before, she has to stop now to take care of her child.

I've often thought that abuse is sometimes an act of momentary stupidity that results in lifelong damage to the child. We've now compounded the damage by leaving the child and mother with no resources. Often, in my experience, the incarcerated perpetrator likely poses no risk to children in the future. Wouldn't it have been better for everyone if we kept the dad out of jail and sentenced him to providing child support for the rest of his life? Perhaps the whole family would be better off.

## About Joshua

Joshua, son of Peter and Rebecca, died just short of his third month of life. At his autopsy, the medical examiner found evidence of significant head trauma. The medical examiner said Joshua died from shaken baby syndrome. During his short life, Joshua had been the victim of at least two, if not three, episodes of inflicted head injury.

The investigation into Joshua's death stalled after a time, as so many of these investigations do. Dead baby cases rarely have a witness, rarely have forensic scene evidence, never have a victim statement, and, unless there is a confession or clear evidence that the fatal injury could only have occurred while the baby was in the care of a particular person, no prime suspect.

So it was with Joshua. No doubt Joshua had been killed. No doubt one of his parents had killed him. His extensive injuries were not accidental and only Rebecca and Peter took care of him. Unfortunately, based solely on the medical evidence, there was no way to say which of the two had done it.

Peter told the police that he and Joshua were home alone. Rebecca had started back to work that very day. Peter said he heard a noise from the infant monitor in Joshua's room. It sounded like Joshua was choking. He rushed into the room and found Joshua unresponsive, his arms and legs flailing. It looked to Peter as if Joshua was having another seizure just like the one he had a month earlier. Perter said that in trying to arouse Joshua he gently shook him, but it didn't help. Peter then put Joshua in the car and rushed him to the nearby doctor's office. In the doctor's office Joshua was limp and unresponsive. From the doctor's office, Joshua was taken by ambulance to the hospital where he was pronounced dead.

No one investigating the case believed that gentle shaking as Peter described could have caused the injuries found at Joshua's autopsy. The problem was not that there was not an identified victim, there was, nor that Peter was not a suspect, he was. The problem was the common law enforcement dilemma of the alternative suspect. One possible scenario was that after Rebecca left for work, Peter caused the fatal head injury that led to Joshua's death. Another possible scenario was that Rebecca had caused the ultimately fatal head injury before going to work and that Joshua had then lain unconscious until Peter found him gasping and near death. Since neither Rebecca nor Peter could be ruled out as a suspect, the case quickly went cold. Sadly, as is often the case, Joshua's death was left unexplained and unavenged, one of an endless litany of beaten and dead babies. Eventually the police stopped investigating, not casually or cynically. But, as other cases took precedence, the memory of Joshua faded.

A year later another son was born to Peter and Rebecca. Because of what had happened to Joshua, this baby was placed into foster care by child protective services. No judge, no child welfare worker would take the chance of leaving this new baby in the home where another child had been killed.

Rebecca might have been able to keep her infant out of foster care if it were clear that Peter had abused Joshua, if it were clear that Rebecca had no culpability in Joshua's death, if it were clear that Rebecca had no prior knowledge that Joshua had been at risk, and finally if Rebecca were willing to separate from Peter. Then, perhaps, she could have kept Daniel. There were too many ifs.

One month after this new infant was placed into foster care and over a year since Joshua had been killed, Peter was watching the news and saw me talking about shaken baby prevention. I talked about what happens to a baby's brain when they are shaken, and demonstrated with a doll what shaking might look like to an observer. Peter later said that the demonstration had suddenly awakened in him the memory that he had indeed shaken Joshua with the same kind of force that I had used with the doll. Peter confessed first to his priest then to the police. After his confession, Peter and Rebecca separated. Rebecca was then able to get her son back. Six months later, Peter was arrested. Nine months after that, he went on trial for manslaughter.

I became aware of Joshua and Peter not because I had seen Joshua, which I hadn't, but because Peter's attorney asked to meet with me to see if I might be willing to help him in preparing his defense for the upcoming trial. I had known this attorney for a number of years. He had always been gracious and respectful, particularly when cross-examining me on the witness stand, something I am always grateful for.

After speaking with Peter's attorney, I agreed to read the case records including the autopsy report and the initial pre-confession and later post-confession police interviews. I was particularly interested in who Peter was and what his story had to say about how and why babies are shaken.

Joshua's autopsy report was straightforward, comprehensive, tragic, and all too familiar. He had old and new hemorrhages on the surface of his massively swollen brain. There were extensive hemorrhages in the back of the eyes, old and new hemorrhages in the neck muscles, and damage to the spinal cord. All of this could only mean violent head and neck rotation as in shaking. The pathologist thought that there had been at least two if not three separate episodes of violent shaking. The rest of the examination, the skin, the bones, the organs (other than the brain) was entirely normal. To any casual observer who might have seen Joshua in the hospital, he would have looked like a healthy three-month-old baby boy. Having seen too many shaken babies, it is always astounding to me how normal some of these babies otherwise look, no bruises, no obvious fractures, nothing to suggest the violence that had been perpetrated on them.

After reviewing the medical, autopsy, and law enforcement records, I told the attorney that I wasn't sure how anything I might say could help Peter. As promised, however, I listened to what he suggested would be his defense. Peter's attorney offered that maybe Peter had shaken the baby the first time out of anxiety while trying to get him to burp and that he had done so not realizing what harm might ensue. He then shook him a second time on the day of his death to try to resuscitate him when he found him unconscious in the crib. The problem with his theory was that the autopsy had shown that the profound injuries on the day of Joshua's death could not have resulted from a gentle shake to resuscitate. The attorney then asked me if I would meet with Peter. I agreed to meet this man who had confessed to killing his child after the investigation had gone cold, who had confessed even though he had been under no pressure to do so.

I was surprised when I met Peter. He was well dressed, well groomed, and well spoken. Every defendant cleans up for trial, but my sense then and since was that the way Peter presented to me that day was how he always presented himself. I saw Peter several times after that meeting, at trial, at his sentencing, after he got out of prison, and always he looked the same. Yet, his eyes, even years later, could not hide the deep sadness he obviously felt over what he had done and what he had lost. Contrite, soft spoken, occasionally tearful, he told me about himself and what he had done to cause his son's death.

Peter described an uneventful childhood and early adulthood. He said that he had a "good upbringing." He had not been abused as a child. He did not drink to excess nor do drugs. He had no previous involvement with law enforcement or with child protective services. As is often the case, it was impossible for me to know how true any of this was. But my sense was that Peter was telling me the truth, and there was no law enforcement or child protective record to contradict him.

He and Rebecca were married when he was 22 and she was 19. They wanted children but their first attempt ended in a miscarriage. They were living out of the country. Peter was working shift work. The miscarriage, the work schedule, the lack of family supports led to tension in the relationship and there was frequent arguing. Peter told me he had a temper. He would sometimes punch walls. After the miscarriage, they went to marriage counseling and things seemed to get better.

When they returned to the States, Rebecca got pregnant a second time and this time gave birth to Joshua, a healthy, vigorous baby boy. Peter told me that Joshua was beautiful. He loved caring for Joshua, at least at first. He particularly loved it when Joshua fell asleep on his chest.

Things were fine for about a month as is often the case with newborns who demand very little other than comfort, food, a dry diaper, and sleep. Peter described Joshua during that first month as a good baby who never really cried. But then, at one month of age, Joshua began to cry. He cried every day usually in the evenings. This was likely normal newborn crying. Some babies cry very little. Some babies cry a lot. Joshua didn't cry during the day and so he was easy for Rebecca to care for. The crying in the evenings however, just when Peter was coming home from work, made it difficult for Peter to enjoy Joshua. The crying upset Peter. It made him anxious. Joshua could likely feel the anxiety, so he cried even more. Both parents found the crying stressful enough that they called their pediatrician on a couple of occasions and were reassured that this was just normal newborn colic. They even took Joshua to the emergency room one evening when the crying seemed particularly bad. Again they were reassured that Joshua was fine.

At two months of age, Joshua received his first set of immunizations. A few days later, he had what Peter described as a seizure. Peter, in his eventual confession, admitted that he had shaken Joshua for the first time some days before the immunizations and the seizure. In all likelihood, it was the residual effect of the head trauma caused by Peter shaking Joshua that brought on the seizure, not the immunizations.

After the seizure, Peter and Rebecca took Joshua to see his pediatrician who referred him to a neurologist. The neurologist felt that the seizure could have been secondary to the immunizations (he didn't know about the shaking), however, he did order a CT scan of the head which was read as normal. As I reviewed the CT scan in preparation for trial, I was surprised to find that it was not normal. There was small amount of blood on the surface of the brain, probably secondary to head trauma from that first shake. Of course Peter was the only one who knew what he had done and he told no one at the time. He also did not, in his own mind, link the shaking to the seizure.

After the seizure, Joshua was even fussier and often inconsolable. Joshua now not only cried but screamed. Though he did not tell Rebecca, Peter was becoming even more uncomfortable caring for Joshua.

Peter went into some detail with me describing what he had done to Joshua. Occasionally, I would stop him to ask for clarifying details, such as exactly how was he holding Joshua, exactly how Joshua's head moved when he was shaken, exactly how Joshua behaved after being shaken. But for the most part Peter simply, if somewhat tearfully, told me the whole story.

The first time Peter shook Joshua they were alone at home. Rebecca had gone out to the store. Joshua started to cry. He cried loudly. He cried as if he were in pain. He cried incessantly. Peter held him. He walked with him. He bounced him on his knee and on his shoulder. No matter what Peter did, Joshua would not stop crying.

Peter tried everything he could think of. He didn't know what else to do. Finally in his exasperation, in his frustration, likely in his anger, he shook Joshua. He was holding Joshua under the arms with his hands squeezing the chest. He shook him, Peter told me, for a couple of seconds. This seems like a short time but in two seconds the head of a baby can rotate back and forth as many as six times. This is six times that the brain is violently crashing, first into the back of the skull and then into the front. After his eventual confession, Peter told Rebecca that he had "vented," apparently meaning he vented his frustration on Joshua by shaking him until Joshua indeed stopped crying.

Unfortunately, shaking works, it does stop the crying. It does so by causing a concussion or worse. This it did to Joshua, who appeared to then fall asleep on Peter's chest, just the way Peter loved him to do.

The shaking was not enough to kill Joshua, but it was enough to cause some injury to the brain and bleeding on the surface of the brain. It was this injury that led to the seizure. It was this injury that caused the few drops of blood I saw on the CT scan.

If Joshua had never been shaken again, he probably would have recovered. He may have developed a seizure disorder. He may have had developmental problems, maybe learning disabilities, but he would not have died. It was the final shake, the last violent shake that killed Joshua.

The first shake did have one terrible consequence. Because of the head trauma, Joshua was even more irritable. He cried even more, every night for hours at a time. Babies do generally soothe better with their mothers. It's no one's fault. It's just the way babies work. But now the crying was worse and the effect of that crying on Peter was inevitably and horribly tragic for Joshua.

The day of Joshua's death Rebecca had gone back to work for the first time. Peter and Joshua were again alone in the house. Peter told me that he heard Joshua gasping in his crib and rushed in to find him, seemingly unconscious, flailing his arms and legs. He looked to Peter like he was having another seizure. Peter took Joshua out of the crib and gave him a shake to try to arouse him. When that didn't work, Peter put Joshua in the car and drove to the doctor's office. From there, Joshua was taken by ambulance to the local hospital where he was pronounced dead.

This sequence of events, as told by Peter, initially to the police and later to me, loss of consciousness followed by a shake to resuscitate, is usually the exact opposite of what really happens. From numerous confessions I have heard, what really happens is that the baby is crying, the perpetrator shakes the baby, and then unconsciousness follows. Peter could not then nor really ever, admit to that last violent shake. He always held that he shook Joshua the last time not out of frustration but to try to get him to come around. Although Peter could never admit this to himself, much less to others, the autopsy showed such severe fresh injuries that this sequence, a shake followed by unconsciousness, is certainly what happened.

Peter had not confessed to what he had done to Joshua when first interviewed by the police. Perhaps he had repressed it. Perhaps he had just lied. But he told no one and things would have stayed that way forever except that he saw me on TV demonstrating how a baby is shaken. Peter told me that when he saw this he immediately realized what he had done. Although he felt that he had not shaken Joshua as hard as I had demonstrated on the news, he still recognized that he had shaken Joshua and that it was this that had caused his death. He said that the realization was like a message from God. He said that he prayed to God and God told him what to do. Peter told his pastor, several of his colleagues, his boss, Rebecca, then the police and finally me. He told me that he felt as if God had forgiven him but that he could not forgive himself. He told the detective that it was funny how you can repress things and then all of a sudden it can come back to you.

Why had Peter shaken Joshua? He wanted to be a good father, not just a good father but *the best* father. More important, he wanted to be *seen* as the best father, not only by Rebecca but by Joshua himself. He felt intensely disappointed in himself when he could not get Joshua to stop crying. He felt frustrated and angry with himself. He denied any anger or frustration with Joshua, although he did tell the police that he shook Joshua "out of anger."

Peter admitted being frustrated and even angry just prior to the first shake, not at Joshua but at himself for his incompetence, his impotence, his inability to sooth Joshua. He felt not just incompetence and frustration but jealousy, jealousy that Joshua would sooth for Rebecca but not for him. Sometimes Rebecca would take Joshua from him because he could not get Joshua to stop crying. This made him feel even worse. Although he was loathe admitting it, Rebecca made him angry when she took Joshua from him.

The defense argument at Peter's trial was multipronged. Shaken baby prevention and education had not started in the United States until right around Joshua's death and even later in Maine. Maybe what happened wasn't Peter's fault since he did not know it was so harmful to shake a baby. Another argument the defense offered was that Joshua had no other injuries. There was no blow or blows to the head, there were no fractures or bruises. Peter's attorney suggested that this meant that there was no intent on Peter's part to harm Joshua, that Peter had not acted recklessly or with the criminal negligence. Another argument at trial was that the first shake occurred because Peter was trying to get Joshua to burp and the second was to get him to stop seizing.

When it came time for me to testify on behalf of Peter, I could not say that what had been done to Joshua was anything other than abuse. I don't know anything about intent, then or now, but I did testify that I believed Peter acted recklessly.

I testified about shaken baby education and when it started in Maine. I testified about the absence of other injuries. I spoke about Peter, his immaturity, his frustration over his own incompetence. I said both on direct questioning by Peter's attorney and in cross-examination by the prosecutor that the shaking was violent and grossly inappropriate, so much so that any observer of the shaking would be horrified at what they saw. I am not sure my testimony helped the defense. In retrospect, I wondered if calling me as a defense witness was the attorney's trying to send a message to the judge and jury that I didn't think Peter was a bad person. Certainly that was true. But it is not just bad people who do bad things. I felt some sympathy for Peter. I knew from seeing him both before and after he was in prison that no conviction, no sentence could possibly punish him more than he would punish himself for the rest of his life.

Peter was convicted of manslaughter. I testified for Peter at his sentencing at his request. As at trial, I spoke of the violence Joshua had experienced in his short life. I spoke about the tragedy of Joshua's death, about how many people had suffered, Rebecca, Joshua's grandparents, other relatives, and friends. I also spoke about Peter himself, his remorse, his shame, and his ultimate contrition. Rebecca also spoke in defense of Peter at his sentencing. She had their infant son, then a year old, with her. It was the last time Peter would ever see him.

In the end, Peter was sentenced to 10 years in prison, five of which were suspended. He did not appeal his conviction or his sentence. He served 28 months, first in a maximum security prison then in a minimum security facility. After that, he was on probation for the remainder of the 10-year sentence. Prison inmates hate child abusers more than anyone else. Peter never told me what prison was like for him and I never asked.

Some years later, Peter and I stood at a national shaken baby conference in front of a standing room only audience of child abuse professionals and parents of shaken babies. We were there because Peter, still on probation but out of prison, contacted me and asked if there was anything he could do to help prevent what he had done from happening to another baby. I immediately thought of that conference. I thought we could present the story of how Joshua had died. I would talk about the medical evidence. Peter would talk about what had happened and, more important, why it had happened.

This conference, the only one of its kind, draws many hundreds of professionals who investigate shaken baby syndrome, including medical professionals, law enforcement, child protective professionals, prosecutors, and even defense attorneys. It also functions as a support network for parents and their often badly head injured babies. Scattered through our audience were not only professionals but parents, not those who had abused the babies, but those who were also victims of sometimes husbands, sometimes partners, sometimes babysitters who had assaulted their infant. There were fathers, mothers, and of course babies, some in specially equipped wheel chairs, paralyzed, blind, deaf, and profoundly cognitively damaged.

Some in the audience would be interested in what Peter might say. Some would be angry, even openly hostile. No one in the audience was in the mood to be lied to. They would not let Peter minimize what he had done. They would offer no forgiveness or sympathy.

I told the audience what injuries Joshua had suffered. I spoke about the likely mechanism and the fact that Joshua had been shaken at least two times.

Peter spoke about his immaturity, about how maybe if there had been some help, some education, some support, Joshua would be alive today. He said that he wished he knew then what normal newborn crying meant, that it didn't mean that the baby had a temper or was angry, that it didn't mean that he was a failure as a parent. He talked about how his expectations for himself as a husband and father had set him up for failure.

Peter told the audience that indeed he had shaken Joshua, not one time, not two times, but three times in all. The first two times he had shaken him out of frustration. But he could not, would not, admit that the last shake was violent enough to cause Joshua's death.

Several audience members expressed reservation, even disbelief at what Peter was saying about that final day. Several parents told Peter that what he had done was unforgivable.

Peter had lost both of his children and his wife. After the trial, Rebecca divorced him. Even if she still loved him there was no way she could stay with the man who had killed her son.

There is another story here, equally sad, equally tragic. Should Peter have been allowed to see his surviving son? I have heard child welfare professionals say perpetrators of fatal child abuse should have no contact ever with their surviving children. When I ask them why, they say it's to protect the child. But let us be clear what we are really talking about here. We are not talking about protecting children from violence in the future. Appropriately supervised contact for someone like Peter would not put his infant at risk. What we are talking about here is retribution, about punishing Peter for what he had done to Joshua and for what he had taken away from Rebecca. I can understand all of that. I can understand how, for some professionals, preventing Peter from seeing his surviving child seemed fair and just, even satisfying. Yet it all seems so gray to me. Even after 30 years of child abuse work, of 30 years of dead and battered babies, of perpetrators, of victims, I still don't know the right answer.

I think about Peter often, not just because he came to that conference with me but about what his story says, not only about child abuse fatality but about crime and punishment. I believe Peter was justly convicted and, although many might think his sentence too lenient, I believe his sentence was equally just. There are crimes against children where no sentence is too long, where even life in prison is not long enough. I don't believe it was ever Peter's intent to kill Joshua. But for Joshua and Rebecca, Peter's intent did not matter in the least.

Peter was not a violent criminal. One could argue, and Peter would agree, that he had a temper. But was Peter likely to ever again harm a child? I want to believe not. There are individuals who I know will harm a child again, who should never ever be alone with a child. For whatever reason, maybe the contrition, the remorse, or even because I'm just trying to preserve some hope in the face of devastating child abuse, I have to believe that Peter was not one of these individuals.

As in most cases like Joshua's, there were any numbers of opportunities to prevent his death. They probably started with whatever led him to develop an anger problem, to misattribute normal crying in Joshua to a temper, to dangerously believe that Joshua's crying reflected badly on him rather than being just a normal expression of infancy. An astute nurse or physician might have seen behavior suggesting risk and been able to intervene. Joshua did cry a lot. There were phone calls to the doctor's office and at least one hospital visit because of the crying. These were clear warnings that Joshua's crying was causing stress for the family. Even later still when Joshua developed the seizure, subtle evidence of trauma was missed on the CT scan. After that it was too late.

Peter did not have to attend that conference with me. He did not have to stand in front of that hostile audience listening to the raw truth of what they thought of him. Peter, through tears, acknowledged that but for his actions, his son would be alive today, he would still be married to Rebecca, and he would be seeing his surviving son. It was one of the bravest things I have ever seen.

Peter and I exchanged a few e-mails after the conference. Then we lost touch. I did learn that he had started dating. I think he was working but he only had a high school diploma and he was now a convicted felon. In my heart of hearts, I have always wished him well.

But what of Rebecca? What of her unendurable grief? What can we learn from parents like her who, through no fault of their own, lose everything? Though I can't tell Rebecca's story, I can, later in this book, tell the stories of Jake's mother Pam and of Lincoln's father Benjy.

Not all cases of child abuse death present like Joshua's, not all perpetrators are seemingly low risk. Many, if not most cases, involve perpetrators with multiple risk factors including substance abuse, domestic violence, child abuse in their own childhood, and law enforcement involvement. The story of Justice tells an entirely different tale of family dysfunction, violence, death, and the failure of the child protective safety net.

## CHAPTER SIX

# Failure to Protect: The Taking of Justice

No one in the field of child welfare wants to judge a family as hopeless, undeserving of even the effort of family preservation or reunification services. Yet, sometimes our very hope for preserving or reunifying a family puts a child at lethal risk.

Anyone who has participated in case reviews of how and why children die from abuse soon arrives at the sickening conclusion that the stories are always the same. The same risk factors are present. The same warning signs are present. The same mistakes happen, again and again. Unfortunately, we have not yet figured out how to protect children from severe, often fatal abuse at the hands of high-risk parents.

In 1987, Doctor David Jones, a psychiatrist in the United Kingdom, published a paper that was provocatively titled "The Untreatable Family" (Jones 1987). Jones defined the untreatable family as one where it is, and may forever be, unsafe for an abused child to live. His contention flew in the face of family preservation and family reunifications advocates.

Jones noted that, if a child is physically abused, there is a significant chance of further abuse if left in the same home. Worse still, some families do not respond to intervention to prevent such further abuse. Some of the factors predictive of a poor outcome in his review were severe abuse in the parent's childhood, persistent denial of abusive behavior, refusal to accept help, severe personality disorder, and substance abuse. All this is made worse if a parent lacks empathy for his or her child. He also noted that severe abuse such as fractures, burns, and premeditated infliction of pain are more likely to prove untreatable. Jones closed his review by suggesting that, if such "untreatable" families can be identified, children can be saved from further abuse as long as they do not remain with those families.

In *The Book of David: How Preserving Families Can Cost Children's Lives*, Richard Gelles, a sociology professor at the University of Pennsylvania, described the tragic case of David, an infant murdered by his mother after multiple involvements with the child welfare system (Gelles 1996). Gelles blamed David's death on the doctrine that social service agencies are required "to make reasonable efforts" to keep an abused child with their parents or, if removed, to reunite the family as soon as possible. He condemned the commonly held belief that children are nearly always better off with their parents if keeping them with their parents puts them at further risk of abuse. He rejected the policy of what he felt was uncritical family preservation and reunification. He argued that child safety rather than family preservation should be the first priority of the child welfare system. He also suggested that more accurate risk assessment tools are needed to help child welfare professionals determine which families pose the greatest risk.

Astonishingly, in the United States, the lifetime prevalence (through age 17) of a child being investigated by the child welfare system is 37 percent (Hyunil et al. 2017). This means that by the time children reach their 18th birthday, fully a third will have been the subject of a child protective investigation. Although it is true that only 22 percent of investigated cases are substantiated, it is also true that most children, who are investigated for abuse, even if not substantiated, later suffer from a variety of negative outcomes. These outcomes can include further abuse, even death.

Eileen Munro, from the London School of Economics, analyzed all child abuse inquiry reports published in Britain from 1973 to 1994 (Munro 1999). During that time frame, there were 45 inquiries into how professionals had handled a child abuse investigation where the later outcome was the death of a child at the hands of a parent.

She found that professionals based their assessment of risk on a narrow range of readily available information. They often ignored information known to other professionals, easily accepted the often dishonest report of family members, and failed to change their opinion when new contradictory information became available. Munro felt that errors in professional decision making are not random but are predictable. If there is a continuum from objective, predictive tools to subjective, intuitive reasoning, Munro argue that both should be used. Intuitive judgement should be treated as a hypothesis that is then tested in a rigorous and systematic manner.

---

### Rachel Berger MD, MPH, Pittsburgh, Pennsylvania

As a researcher, I find the child protective system frustrating. The system does not use evidence to drive policy and practice. This became clear to me when I served as the research lead for the Commission to Eliminate Child Abuse and Neglect Fatalities (Commission to Eliminate Child Abuse and Neglect Fatalities 2016). As commission members traveled around the country, we would hear almost daily reports of child abuse fatalities. Over and over we saw the same errors in decision making. Often these errors would directly lead to a preventable death. I thought about putting a book together of all the news feeds from 2014 child maltreatment deaths. The stories were the same. Only the names changed.

I can't count the number of times I read about an infant seen who had been seen by CPS for bruising, then left in the home to die. In the field of child abuse pediatrics, we know that bruising in nonmobile infants is a strong indicator of future life-threatening risk.

We wouldn't allow what happens in the child protection system to happen in the health-care system. We would not practice medicine in the 21st century the way it was practiced in the 20th century. We try to learn from our mistakes.

Yet, in child welfare, the same mistakes recur. We saw significant push-back by the CPS system over recommendations to develop guidelines. In medicine, we know that guidelines lead to better outcomes.

Another problem I have seen repeatedly is the lack of close ongoing collaboration between child abuse pediatricians and the CPS system. I once saw a child with a fracture that I thought was highly suspicious for abuse. The CPS worker wondered if maybe the baby had fallen off the bed, even though the parents never offered such a fall as an explanation for the injury. Even if the baby had fallen from the bed, it would not have explained that particular fracture. On their own, the worker decided that a fall must have happened and returned the child to the family without consulting with me first.

I believe that one of the keys to decreasing morbidity and mortality from child abuse is improving collaboration between child abuse pediatricians and CPS for all cases of suspected physical abuse in children under 2 or 3 years of age. I believe this will save lives.

In another case, a child who had been seen many times by child protective services for neglect was finally removed from her home. When she came in to see us after her removal, she had old and new belt marks all over her body. Even though CPS had been involved for years, this child had not once been examined for injuries.

I think what happens sometimes is that workers become inured to what they see. They see deplorable conditions every day. They see families with intimate partner violence and drug use. They see unsafe living conditions. They can't remove all of these children so they become blind to the dangers.

CPS caseworkers want to do the right thing. They enter the field because they want to help children. But they are inexperienced, undertrained, often poorly supervised, and overwhelmed by the work load. On top of that, the system is woefully underfunded. At every turn, CPS is castigated by the press and the public either for over-calling abuse or for under-calling it, for removing too many children or not enough.

The CPS office in our county though has a lot of strengths. The main reason is that we talk to each other. We work together. They paid us to imbed a nurse in each of their offices to make sure children in their care got appropriate medical care. Together we are working toward evidence-based child protective decision making. Every month, we go to their offices for what we call "lunch and learn" and teach the caseworkers about health care-related issues. I am sure there are other great models of collaboration, but this one seems to work for us.

### Carole Jenny, MD, MBA, Seattle, Washington

In Seattle, the police are the only ones who can take emergency custody of an abused child. In one case of mine, a child had horrific injuries. A police officer came in and said to me, "Well, a lot of children hurt themselves. My child fell and broke his collarbone. This can happen accidentally." I told him that this child had multiple severe injuries. I told him the child was abused and needed protection. He said, "I don't think that he's in any danger."

It's frustrating to me that someone who knows nothing about child abuse, who has had no training in child abuse, and who has no experience with injuries other that what happens to their own child in play, has that kind of decision-making power.

In this case, I called his sergeant. The sergeant said he would look into it but nothing happened. Then I tried to call the special assault detective unit but I couldn't reach anyone. By then it was late in the night and I had already been on the phone for a couple of hours. Finally, I called the prosecutor in the district attorney's office who deals with special assault cases. She called the police and got the patrol officer's call reversed.

What if this case had been managed by a doctor who was less knowledgeable and experienced then me? Likely this child would have been returned to the home where he had been abused. It is all very frustrating.

### Allison M. Jackson, MD, MPH, Washington, D.C.

Child protective services is obviously an overwhelmed system. There is inconsistent decision making and there is under-utilization of the expertise of medical child abuse teams like ours. Locally though, we are fortunate to have a multidisciplinary team for case review that includes child protective services.

There are still children who slip through the cracks. I sometimes hear from a worker, "It was only one injury." They don't always dig deeper into the family history or look in the case files for other incidents of abuse. If they had, they might have found out that the child had been repeatedly beaten.

I once saw twin babies, both of whom had multiple fractures. As I spoke to the mother, I asked about her own experiences as a child. She told me she had been sexually abused. She wouldn't tell me by whom. When I asked her if she ever told anyone, ever got any help, she dryly told me that she was kicked out of the house when she told her mother. At the age of 15, she was on her own.

Of course, her twins were removed from her care and she was only allowed supervised visits. Even though she had been the one who had abused the children, I felt sympathy for her. I wondered whether the outcome for her and her infants would have been different had she had been evaluated and treated by my team when she was abused as a teenager.

### Richard D. Krugman, MD, Aurora, Colorado

I think our child welfare system in the United States was in a horrible shape in the 1980s and 1990s. That's when we published the U.S. Advisory Board report that described child abuse as a public health emergency (U.S. Advisory Board on Child Abuse and Neglect 1990).

I'm actually impressed now 25 years later. I think the system here in Colorado is much better than it was.

I still don't think our child welfare system is where it needs to be. I think not looking at practice quality and outcomes prevents child welfare, law enforcement, and civil and criminal courts from ever knowing if they are effective. Child abuse policy is currently made on the basis of scandal, not data.

If you read the original works of Henry Kempe and Ray Helfer, they knew how to deal with the problem of child abuse. These early pioneers were very effective in helping individual abusive and neglectful families. But we haven't figured out how to take what we know works for a hundred children and families and make it work for the entire country.

### Kenneth W. Feldman, MD, Seattle, Washington

One of our ICU (Intensive Care Unit) doctors was once so incensed by a case that he went to the legislature and got a law passed. The law said that if a doctor feels that a child is in imminent danger of harm, CPS has to take it to court unless they can prove that the child is safe. Prior to that, the law required that CPS prove the child is in danger. Now, if we feel a child is unsafe, CPS has to prove they are safe.

I think we have pretty good relationships with child protective services. We have worked together for a long time. Whenever we have a serious case, we conference directly with CPS and law enforcement and make sure they understand the medical facts of the case. They make sure we understand the investigative aspects of the case. Their investigations often reveal previously unsuspected risk factors and provide valuable scene injury reconstruction.

### Howard Dubowitz, MD, MS, Baltimore, Maryland

What is most distressing for me looking back is that at the community and societal levels, we have not made enough progress in improving the lives of our children. I've been working in Sweden and am envious of how Sweden is a decent place for children to live. I've been working in West Baltimore for over 30 years and it remains a difficult place to live for too many children.

Working with CPS is often frustrating. I am sympathetic to the fact that they have a very tough job. But one case in family court stands out for me. I was quite sure that an infant had been badly abused and was at serious risk of further abuse if returned to the parents. CPS placed the child with his grandparents. A few weeks later, the court decided to return the baby to the parents. I am quite cautious about sticking my neck out in these situations, but I remember thinking at the time that if anything happens to this baby, I am going to go to the media. Sure enough, within a day of returning home, the infant was killed. I never did go to the media.

### Marcellina Mian, MDCM, MPHE, Qatar

It's not just the child welfare system that fails children. I once reviewed a case where a young girl was living with her father because her mother had a history of drug abuse. By report, he seemed reliable and caring. He had remarried and the child was visiting her mother saying that the stepmother was being mean to her. Her mother had seen bruises and the young girl said the stepmother had caused them. Her mother brought her to her family doctor who was also the doctor for the father and his wife. This doctor could not believe that either of them would harm the little girl. So he tested her for a bleeding disorder. Even though the tests came back normal, the doctor did not make a report to CPS. The following weekend, the stepmother killed the little girl.

I used to call some families "the lovelies." They are lovely in every way except that their child has inflicted injuries. It's important for professionals to recognize that when they see "the lovelies" they are only seeing someone's best public face. They really don't know what is going on behind closed doors.

### Desmond K. Runyan, MD, DrPH, Denver, Colorado

In another state, a hospital-based child protective team took child protective services to court because they were unhappy with how cases were being handled. After they won the court case, CPS stopped referring children to them. They won the battle but lost the war. I decided that having an adversarial relationship with CPS was not helpful to children and I was not going to do that.

Our relationship with child protective services is pretty positive. We now train every social worker in the state of Colorado. We try very hard to keep communication open.

## About Justice

It breaks my heart that, despite all the trainings we do about abusive injuries to doctors, nurses, home visitors, and child welfare workers, babies still fall through the cracks. So many professionals failed Justice, it is almost beyond reckoning.

Justice was taken to see his doctor when he was one-month-old because of a swollen leg. X-rays showed a break across the femur (thigh bone). His parents told the doctor that the baby had fallen from dad's lap and that the leg must have broken during the fall. Unfortunately, for whatever reason, the doctor believed the story of an accidental injury even though such a fall could not have caused that particular fracture. A report was never made to child protective services, not by the doctor or the doctor's staff, not by the radiologist or the radiologist's staff, and not by the orthopedist or the orthopedist's staff. Even if these providers thought it likely that the injury was accidental, there was no way they could have said it was definitely not abuse. The correct response should have been a report to child protective services.

Had a report been made and had CPS investigated, they would have found a family rife with risk factors. Both parents had been abused as children, had been in the foster care system, and the baby's father had a history of violence.

A few weeks later, Justice was seen by another medical provider for a well-child check and bruising was seen on his face. When asked, the mother suggested that maybe an older sibling had bruised the baby. The provider sent the baby for blood work to rule out a bleeding disorder and, despite these tests being normal, did nothing further. It was likely, though not known for certain, that this provider knew of the prior fracture. Again no report was made to CPS. The bruising had also been seen by a visiting nurse and daycare providers. Yet again, no one reported this to CPS.

Four days before he died, Justice was seen by a child protective worker for concerns about the family unrelated to Justice. The family told the worker about the fracture. They did not tell the worker about the bruising, but neither did the worker ask if there had been any bruising. The worker concluded that the home was safe.

If a child abuse pediatrician had been called at any time about any of the injuries Justice had sustained before he died, they would have recommended Justice be hospitalized immediately for an abuse evaluation. On the day of his death, Justice was finally seen by a child abuse pediatrician but by then it was too late. Justice was in the hospital with a lethal head injury. He also had multiple fractures throughout his body.

Eventually, Justice's father pled guilty to causing his son's death by shaking him. He also confessed that the fall had never happened, that he had broken Justice's leg out of frustration. He received a lengthy prison sentence.

What went wrong in this case? Why was Justice not saved? Multiple mandated reporters failed to report either of the two sentinel injuries

(injuries that predict later more serious abuse), the broken bone and the fracture. None of the providers talked to each other, so no one knew the whole story. In this case, primary prevention strategies such as home visitation did not work, at least in part, because the family was so dysfunctional and high risk.

A chilling question remains. If Justice had not sustained that final lethal injury, would we have ever known about his abuse? If the answer is no, how many other children are profoundly abused and never recognized. How many other children later develop lifelong disabilities from their unrecognized and untreated abuse?

## About Chelsea

Although this chapter focuses on nonmedical errors in decision making, it is important to remember that the child welfare system cannot be held responsible for a death or serious injury if the sentinels whose responsibility it is to identify and report abuse fail in their job.

Vickie and Patrick took their three-month-old daughter Chelsea to see her doctor because she was vomiting. They told the doctor, in passing, that Chelsea seemed to bruise easily when held. The doctor saw a bruise on the right side of her jaw. The parents seemed likeable enough so his suspicion for child abuse was low. Even so, he included child abuse in his written note as a possible diagnosis along with accidental injury and bleeding disorder.

If the doctor had seriously considered child abuse as a possible cause for the bruising, the next step should have been to report to CPS and admit Chelsea to the hospital for a more complete evaluation. Unfortunately for Chelsea, neither was done. Chelsea was sent home with her parents who were told to return should the bruising occur again. This seemingly trivial bruising signaled the beginning of a tragic cascade of misery for Chelsea.

Unknown to the doctor, Patrick had started caring for Chelsea a month earlier when Vickie went back to work. He found Chelsea's crying stressful. At the time of his eventual confession, Patrick told the police that he had stifled Chelsea's cries by grabbing her face and covering her mouth. This is what had caused the bruise seen by the doctor.

Four days after the visit to the doctor's office, Patrick slapped Chelsea across the face. He told Vickie who told her supervisor at the nursing home where she worked. Neither told anyone else.

Two weeks later, while Vickie was at work, Patrick took Chelsea to the emergency department because she had suddenly become unconscious. He told the staff that she was crying in his arms and lunged back. She hit her head on the table and seemed stunned. Her eyes rolled back in her head. At the hospital, Chelsea seemed fine.

After hearing from Vickie that Patrick and Chelsea were at the hospital, Vickie's supervisor at the nursing home called the hospital and told the emergency room nurse that she had concerns about the baby. She told them that Vickie had told her that Patrick had hit Chelsea.

This information was relayed to the treating physician. Chelsea's examination was normal and both parents (Vickie arrived later) seemed appropriate. The nurse and the physician discussed the call between themselves. They then discharged Chelsea to her parents without notifying anyone, not child protective services, not even Chelsea's doctor. If Chelsea's doctor, who knew about the prior bruise, had been called, perhaps he would have called CPS. A copy of the hospital record with documentation of the phone call was mailed to the doctor. Later the doctor could not recall if he ever saw that report.

During his later confession to the police, Patrick described what really happened that day. Chelsea had been crying. Nothing Patrick could do would calm her. In his increasing agitation, he struck her across the back of her head with an open hand. This did stop her crying. It also stunned her. Her eyes briefly rolled back into her head.

One week after the emergency room visit, Patrick slapped Chelsea, now almost four months old, twice in the face. This caused a bloody nose and bruising around both eyes. He told Vickie that Chelsea had fallen from her bouncy chair.

One week after that he viciously struck her in the head with a closed fist. She immediately lost consciousness. This time she did not wake up. Fearing the worst, he took her to the hospital. He told the hospital staff, the same hospital staff that had seen them before, that Chelsea had struck her head on the crib rail as she rolled over. This time no one believed him.

Chelsea had a skull fracture, bruising and swelling of her brain, hemorrhages in the back of her eyes, and a torn liver. She was in the hospital for two months.

Patrick pled guilty to assault and was sent to prison. Chelsea was taken into foster care then adopted. She is now blind, deaf, nonverbal, and wheelchair bound.

What went wrong in this case? The primary care provider, despite suspicion of possible abuse, did not call child protective services. During the first hospital visit, the concerns raised by the nursing home supervisor were not taken seriously. If they had been, child protective services would have been called. At the very least, there should have been discussion between the emergency room doctor and the primary care provider about the visit. If such discussion had occurred, perhaps a report would then have been made to child protective services, but, as can be seen from other cases in this chapter, perhaps even then Chelsea would not have been saved from her devastating brain injury.

## About John

Luckily, some child welfare mistakes do not end badly.

John came to the hospital when he was one-month-old with a broken leg. His x-ray revealed that his right femur (thigh bone) was badly broken. The initial history from the parents to the CPS worker and the detective was that they were sitting on opposite ends of the couch. John was lying between them on a pillow. It was 1 A.M. His dad, Anthony, was playing Call of Duty on the computer. His mother Samantha was eating. John somehow slipped and his dad grabbed his leg. John did not cry. An hour later, John was screaming in his bed. His parents took him to the hospital where he was admitted for treatment of the broken leg and for a child abuse evaluation.

When I went into the room to talk to the parents, the CPS worker and detective were finishing up their interviews. I did not like the content or the tone of the interviews. The detective seemed to be pulling random questions out of the air rather than systematically exploring the story. The CPS worker was very sympathetic to the distraught dad. At one point she actually told him not to beat himself up over an accident. Clearly, the CPS worker had already made her mind up that the broken leg was an accident. The detective seemed out of his depth. I was left with an uneasy feeling even before I had started my own assessment of the injury.

I first spoke with Samantha. My initial and ongoing impression of her was of a sort of apathy. When discussing the broken leg, and even later when talking about the additional injuries we discovered, she showed no emotion. One could argue that her lack of emotion was because of shock, but she continued to show little to no emotion even weeks later when, presumably, the initial shock should have worn off.

Samantha told me that they had all been together on the couch. She was sitting on the left, the baby was in the middle on a pillow, and Anthony on the right playing his video game.

I don't like dads or boyfriends playing violent video games while caring for a baby, not because of the game's effect on the baby, but because of the game's effect on the adult. Imagine a crying baby in that environment. It would be all too easy to lash out, shoot the enemy, slap the baby.

Samantha told me that John was fussing and then he seemed to slip. Anthony grabbed the leg to stop him from falling. John did not cry out but continued to fuss. Anthony started feeding him but Samantha took over and sent Anthony to bed because the feeding was not going well. An hour later, John cried out in his bed and they took him to the hospital.

Anthony, in his interview with me, was nervous. He had poor eye contact. He told me that he does get frustrated with the baby but he will walk away. He admitted to a problem with anger inherited from his father who had "terrible anger issues."

His story of what happened to John was just enough different from Samantha's to concern me. They were all three on the couch. The baby was on the pillow between them. Samantha said the baby was sideways head toward Anthony. Anthony said the baby's head was toward Samantha. He repeated the story of the almost fall and said he may have grabbed the leg too hard but not intentionally. John though did not cry and Anthony did not hear or feel a pop which often accompanies a major bone break in a baby. He fed the baby and then went to bed. He denied being sent to bed or having the baby taken from him by Samantha.

What was I to make of this? Was it possible that a one-month-old baby could roll from a pillow and have his leg grabbed by his father to prevent a fall? Were the forces involved sufficient to cause the break? And what was I to make of the discrepancies? All of these questions were superimposed on my uneasiness with the obvious quick conclusion of the CPS worker that this was an accident.

Later, when the rest of our screening x-rays were done, another fracture was discovered involving the same leg but this one was older and located at the knee joint. While the femur fracture could have possibly occurred the way the dad said, the joint fracture clearly was from a different injury at a different time. Now there was compelling evidence that John had been injured on more than one occasion.

When I told the CPS worker about the second injury and my opinion that the baby had been abused, she clearly did not accept my conclusion. She said she would talk to her supervisor. She later called me and said that they had decided that the baby was safe going home with both parents with the worker checking in on them a couple times a week. I called the supervisor who told me that the worker thought that both injuries had happened at the same time and were consistent with an accident. The worker told her supervisor that I had said that it was possible that both injuries had happened at the same time. This was not what I had said at all. Thankfully, the supervisor and I agreed that the social worker knew nothing about injury biomechanics. The supervisor told the worker to return to the hospital to tell the parents that the child would not be going home with them.

When I saw the worker in the hospital later, she was clearly unhappy with me. Better that, I thought, than a dead baby. The conversation we had together with the parents was even more troubling. She told them that I was responsible for the decision to not send the baby home with them, a decision she did not agree with. The worker kept asking me about other possibilities such as brittle bone disease, vitamin deficiency, and prematurity. Finally, after answering some of these questions respectfully, my frustration got the better of me and I told her that she was supposed to be a child protective worker not a defense attorney. She stopped talking to me after that. Later a different worker was assigned to the case.

When I saw John in follow-up a few weeks later with his mother and grandmother, they still were not convinced that the injuries were inflicted. I hear over and over again from a parent that a child could not have been abused because this parent knows the other parent and knows that they could never hurt a child. My response is always the same, "The only thing you know for sure is what you have done. You can never know what someone else has done. You can never know what someone else is capable of." Sometimes that works; often it falls on deaf ears.

In this case they were not convinced. They even argued with me that a follow-up set of x-rays, standard in child abuse work, was not necessary because John had not been abused. Their opinion changed, however, when the follow-up x-rays showed four additional fractures. This is why we do follow-up x-rays. Some fractures are difficult to see initially but can be seen one to two weeks later when healing starts.

Finally, if all that was not enough, the new worker told me to take a look at the emergency department record. The father had given four different stories to four different providers in the emergency department. The first was that he heard a pop at some point. The second was that he did not hear a pop but rather that the baby started crying after a diaper change and then would not move the leg. The third was that, during the diaper change, he grabbed the leg and John cried out. Finally, the fourth explanation was that the baby started falling off the pillow while he was changing the diaper.

Why do providers make these kinds of mistakes? The worker had jumped to a conclusion before all the information was in. She had not reviewed the emergency department record as the second worker had. She clearly let her sympathy for the seemingly distraught father cloud her assessment. She only accepted information that confirmed her original impression of an accident rather than modify that impression after new contradictory information was found. Thankfully, we did not send the baby back home with the parents but rather placed the baby with a protective grandmother.

This chapter offers no easy answers, only questions and the sickening sense that serious abuse will happen again and again until we finally get it right.

But while we struggle to find the answer, there remain other victims in these tragedies who are rarely heard from. What of parents, grandparents, other relatives and friends who, through no fault of their own, lose a child to abuse? In an earlier chapter, I spoke of Joshua's mother Rebecca. The next chapter tells the story of two such parents who lost their babies at the hands of another.

## CHAPTER SEVEN

# A Parent's Grief: Pam and Benji

Ask a person on the street about shaken baby syndrome and the typical answer might be that it's not good to shake a baby, that it could damage their brain and even kill them. Some might express disbelief or even anger that someone could do that to an innocent infant.

Ask a child abuse pediatrician about shaken baby syndrome and they will talk about rotational injury and shear forces, about damage to the brain, bones, eyes, and about death.

Ask a law enforcement investigator and they will probably tell you about interviewing techniques and confessions.

A child protective worker will explain about safety planning and child protective court action.

A defense attorney, or one of the few shaken baby deniers who testify for the defense, will talk about an imperfect science or, outrageously, about a scam by the medical professionals who promulgated the myth that shaking kills babies.

A defendant, charged or not, convicted or not, may confess, but more commonly will offer a loud denial. "I didn't do it." "Someone else did it." "It was an accident."

All these individuals and others have been asked about shaken baby syndrome. One group, however, has never been heard from, except in the tightly knit confines of survivor support groups. These are the parents, grandparents, siblings, aunts, uncles, and friends who had nothing to do with what happened, yet who now, through no fault of their own, are also victims.

This chapter is about two of these survivors, Jake's mother Pam and Lincoln's father Benjy.

## About Jake

Prior to his death at age four months, Jake was Pam and David's healthy, happy, and much loved infant son. On the day of his death, David as usual woke him, changed his diaper, and dressed him to go to his babysitter's home. Jake that morning was his usual happy, smiling, curious self. David took him to see Pam in their bedroom. She kissed him and told him she loved him. It would be the last time she would see him alive.

Later that day, Jake was taken to one hospital then another where he eventually died. The cause of Jake's death was massive blunt head trauma. The manner of death, according to the medical examiner, was homicide. Eventually, Jake' babysitter pled guilty to shaking him then slamming him down onto a table.

Pam had started back to work a few months earlier as a medical assistant. Even though Pam and David had carefully screened the sitter, they did not learn until after Jake was killed about the sitter's dark secret. Some years earlier, she had lost custody of her nine-year-old daughter, in part because she had hit her over the head with a frying pan.

## Jake's Mother Pam in Her Own Words

It's almost 19 years now. I remember that day as if it were yesterday. I got a call at work at 11:48 A.M. from the sitter. She yelled into the phone, "Jake, Pam, come now."

When I got to her home, I found a police officer giving CPR to Jake's lifeless little body on the kitchen table. The sitter was standing in the small kitchen area a few feet away from me. All she said was, "Pam, I don't know what happened. He choked on his bottle."

After what felt like an eternity (it was really only five minutes), an ambulance arrived. I was able to go with Jake in the ambulance. I remember hearing "epinephrine STAT!" That was the one time in my life that I wished I knew absolutely nothing about the medical field. As a medical professional and a mother I knew that something was very wrong and that Jake had not just choked on his bottle.

On the way to the hospital, I called my husband to tell him that everything was going to be okay, but that I needed him to meet me at the hospital. Something had happened to Jake. He called his parents and my parents. He didn't want to be dealing with me by myself in that situation, so he called in the reinforcements.

At the hospital, the trauma team took Jake. I was escorted to the back of the hospital to, what I now know was, a crisis room. It was a very small room, about the size of a walk-in closet.

After my husband and family arrived, we waited. Eventually, a nurse came in and asked us what happened to our baby. We told her we had no idea. She turned and walked away.

Later, two men in suits arrived. They were a detective and a child protective worker. They separated David and I for questioning. We had no idea what was going on. We just wanted to see our baby. We didn't know why these questions were being asked.

Jake's family physician came in and took David and I to another room. She told us that she had had Jake baptized because the ER doctors thought he was going to die. After that, we finally were allowed to see him. His little body was hooked up to numerous machines that were keeping him alive.

He was transferred to a pediatric hospital where a neurologist spoke with us. He was very brief. He said that our child had been a victim of child abuse and was likely going to die. We spent the rest of the day with state police, again in separate rooms, only seeing Jake intermittently.

I am grateful for all of the professionals in that immediate time. More than anything else, everyone did their job. I mean that. Nobody missed a beat. The information we were given was limited. We were suspects of course, until all the pieces of the puzzle could be put together. Police were investigating behind the scenes while we were at the hospital. One of the police officers had grabbed the bottle that he had supposedly choked on and took it with him. He was observant enough to know that something wasn't right.

The next morning, we were interviewed by a child abuse doctor who told us our son had been a victim of shaken impact syndrome (Author's note: this was the language in use at the time to describe infants with evidence of shaking and impact. The current clinical term is "abusive head trauma"). He finally gave us the information we needed. We now understood that Jake had been a victim of child abuse and that the evidence was pointing at the babysitter.

Later that day, Jake was removed from life support and died in our arms at 3:55 P.M.

Everyone had been wonderful. Earlier in the day, a nurse had put on a Sesame Street audio tape for Jake to listen to. I've always been taught that the last sense to go is hearing. This caring action meant a lot to me. Before he was disconnected from the life support, we were allowed to do things we would never be able to do again, to bathe him, dress him, and give him his first haircut. We dressed him in his Arizona jeans, Big Bird Bobo sneakers, and Pooh shirt. We were allowed to take footprints like we did when he was born. It's the smallest things not noticed by others, the positives and the negatives, that we held onto.

There was one thing though that happened after he was unplugged that we wished we had been warned about. His extremities began to swell. This will stay with us forever. It was one of the hardest things to watch his little body change.

We had a memorial service for Jake. We didn't have a funeral. We had a celebration of life on the beach. It was one of the coldest May days I can remember, raining and bitterly cold. I couldn't tell you how many people were on the beach with us, maybe 200. The babysitter had just been arrested and charged with Jake's death, so press was there as well.

Some of the people there I knew, some I did not. I could not help but think when I saw people I didn't know, "Did they have a child die, and are they here for some closure to their own pain?" I'll never know, but whatever the reason, the important thing was that they were there.

We had a memorial box with us at the beach. The box was a way of remembering the beautiful things that we had shared and even some of the things we would have shared with him. People had an opportunity to speak about their love for Jake and deposit gifts into the box. The gifts varied from a shell someone found on the beach that morning to a picture of children who Jake might have come to know. At the end of the service as we sang "Something Beautiful," my sister Penny released 40 colored balloons tied with a Pooh bear at the bottom. It floated out of sight. At that moment, it felt as though God was with us, as each of us said goodbye to Jake.

I did eventually try to go back to work as a medical assistant. I lasted three hours. There was a baby crying in the waiting room. I told my boss I couldn't stay and left. I never went back.

Jake has been gone 19 years now. People tell you it gets easier. It doesn't. It gets different. It's a roller coaster. I turned to advocacy rather than let the grief get to me. Prevention has been my focus. But even the prevention work was hard. The grieving process doesn't end, especially when you add in child abuse, when your child didn't die in a car accident or by some fluke illness, when your child died at the hands of someone else.

If an adult dies, you grieve for what was, for the memories. If a child dies, you grieve for what should have been, what might have been. I am not sure of the author's name but the saying I heard many years ago comes to mind, "The saddest words of mouth and pen are these four words: what might have been." How true, especially for those who have lost a child and are left to carry on.

I was very fortunate to have a second child, Wyatt, who just turned 18. I think that this last year was the hardest. Wyatt had his junior prom. Jake should have had his senior prom and he should have graduated.

The sitter has been out of prison for a few years. She served 8 ½ years. At the time of her sentencing, she offered a brief guilty plea. It looked like she was trying to turn to us to say she was sorry, but she didn't. She had plenty of opportunity at her sentencing to say what happened that morning, but she chose not to. She lives in the same community we do. More than once, we have had to leave a store where she was in one aisle and we were in another.

There are so many experiences that bring back the grief. Last summer, at a social event, I saw one of the detectives who had worked on the case. He came up to me, shook my hand and said, "Pam, thanks on behalf of the children. You work tirelessly." That was really cool on the one hand, yet it hurt like hell on the other.

Recently my husband and I were involved in a car accident, and we went to the local police department to fill out a report. A police officer took our report. After a while, he looked at me and said "You're Pam. You're Jake's mom." I said, "Yep, I'm Jake's and Wyatt's mom." He looked me in the eye and said, "I was the first responder."

My husband and I definitely grieve differently. Yet, we held the line together and focused on Wyatt and on prevention. Dave co-taught classes for new dads. That was very therapeutic for him.

Grief is not the same for everyone and it doesn't happen the same way and at the same time for a couple. If I was angry, he was sad. If I was sad, he might have been angry. We had to communicate. We had to talk to each other. Even though we were sometimes in different places, we always talked about it. I really believe that as much as it was love, it was communication that has kept us together.

After Wyatt was born, strangers would come up to me to say how cute he was. Then came the hard part: "Is he your first child?" It is a simple question under normal circumstances, but how do you answer that question when your first-born son was killed? Whenever I was asked that question it felt like a knife had been stuck in my heart and turned a notch. In the beginning I would say, "No." But then people would ask, "How old is your other child?" "Do you have a boy or a girl?" That was even more difficult to deal with. Most of the time, if I said no, people would not ask further. If they did, I would say, "My first son was murdered by his babysitter." This would often leave the questioner with a dropped mouth and tears rolling down their cheeks. I would not sacrifice my feelings for those of a stranger. We now say, "No, our first son is an angel."

It's the "would haves, should haves, and could haves" that continue to haunt us. What if we hadn't left him with her that day, or at all? Things would have been different. That stuff will eat you up. It will absolutely eat you up if you let it. We chose a different path. Education is the key. We turned all of those emotions, all that anger, frustration, and just wanting to lay down and die with him, into prevention. Jake was our sunshine. He was our everything. Our lives had changed. So we worked on prevention.

This never should have happened. Why had it happened? I knew about shaken baby syndrome. I was a medical assistant. I had seen the signs, the black and red posters that say NEVER, NEVER SHAKE A BABY. Funny thing, underneath those big letters there is a little sentence that I never paid much attention to that said "may cause deafness, blindness, learning disabilities, even death."

Babies cry. A baby's crying is equivalent to the sound of a jackhammer. It's what we do when that crying gets to be too much that makes the difference. Put them down. It's okay. It doesn't make you a bad parent. It makes you a damn good parent when you say, "You know what. I love you so much that I am going to put you down before I do something that will change our lives forever." That's key. That's what I love about "The Period of PURPLE Crying" prevention program. It's so down-to-earth and so real. Part of what we did was what I call planting seeds of prevention. Through the years, we did a lot of work in prevention with so many different colleagues, nationally and here in our state.

We started the "Don't Shake Jake" awareness program. We made refrigerator labels that said "Don't Shake Jake." They included a crisis response number for fire, doctor, and police and on the bottom it offered a reminder to "Never shake a baby." All Maine hospitals distributed the labels. We made lapel pins of yellow (color of remembrance) and navy blue (national color of child abuse prevention) with an angel in memory of all the children who have become angels because of child abuse. We also had bumper stickers printed that said "Don't Shake Jake."

We also went to the Maine State Legislature to work on a law compassionately known as Jake's Law. We knew that historically if someone killed a child in Maine they were given very light sentences. I found that absolutely unacceptable. The first key is prevention, but we also felt that the voices of these dead children had to be heard and honored. So Jake's Law was passed and it allowed judges to increase the sentence beyond the usual guidelines if a child under the age of 6 was assaulted or killed.

When we went to our hearing in front of the Criminal Justice Committee, the Maine Civil Liberties Union testified in opposition to Jake's Law. The person who testified said the law would not be a deterrent to child abuse and that we should not increase the penalty. This angered me beyond words. The person speaking had no idea what it feels like to lose a child because of someone else's violence.

The first time Jake's Law was used, I sat in the court room and held the hand of the grandmother of a little girl. Her mother's boyfriend had literally beaten the life out of her. He was now being sentenced. The judge sitting on the bench that day said, "I sentence you to five years but the legislature now mandates that because Chelsea was under the age of 6 when she died and because of the heinous nature of the crime, I sentence you to an additional five years." What I heard and what her grandmother heard was additional time for the person who took the life of her granddaughter. I also heard Chelsea's name. When Jake's sitter was sentenced, Jake's name was never mentioned. Chelsea's voice had been heard. That's the power of not laying down and dying with Jake.

I was actually at a child abuse conference the second time Jake's Law was used. A little girl named Logan had been wrapped in 42 feet of duct tape by her foster mother and had suffocated to death. Her foster mother was convicted and sentenced to 20 years in prison. People were saying "Did you hear? Did you hear? She got 20 years!" I remember smiling the same time as I was crying. Again, a child's voice had been heard.

I know everybody says my baby was beautiful. My baby was absolutely beautiful. He had vibrant, big blueberry eyes. He had just enough hair to say it was there. When I put baby lotion in his hair, his hair would spike up. He was absolutely beautiful. By the time he passed, he had just started to do the coos and the oohs and the real smiles.

We didn't have a lot of money then and my mother-in-law had bought this ugly little red pants suit with a little checkered vest. This was a baby who had jeans and Bobo sneakers. If he was a boy, I wanted him to look like a boy. Yet on Valentine's Day, I brought Jake to get his pictures taken in that little red outfit. Little did I know, that would be the outfit that would become synonymous with Baby Jake in the media and around the state.

He was a colicky baby. He had bouts of crying. I would sing to him a lot. We would rock a lot. We would cry together. But he was my joy. He was absolutely my joy. He was my little blue-eyed angel.

Many times I have asked myself, if I had known what the future would hold, would I have given birth to this angel again. My answer has always been definitely yes. As a new mom you find that when they place your baby in your arms that first time, you have never before felt such love.

## About Lincoln

Lincoln was four months old when he became unresponsive in the care of a babysitter. He died four days later from what was described as severe blunt head trauma and brain injury. His babysitter was convicted of causing Lincoln's death and sentenced to 13 years in prison.

## Lincoln's Father Benjy in His Own Words

Lincoln was totally healthy when he was born. He was breathing on his own. He didn't have to go to the NICU (Newborn Intensive Care Unit) even though he was four weeks premature. Everything was good.

He was our first baby so we were new parents trying to figure it all out. We have had two since and looking back he was a normal newborn. He was a month early, so he needed to be fed a lot at the beginning. He was bottle fed and my wife and I took turns feeding him day and night.

He was developing normally as far as we could tell and as far as we were told. He'd had his three month checkup. He was gaining weight like he was supposed to. He was really small at first. When we took him home from the hospital, he was only five pounds, but then we went in a week later and he was five and a half. When he passed away, he was up to 13 pounds. He was starting to get more interactive. He was smiling and cooing and reaching for things. We had just started him on rice cereal. He slept well, not at first, but once he got a little weight on him he slept through the night. We thought everything was good.

I remember going in his room that day. He was still asleep. I actually remember turning the light on and trying to run over to cover his face so the light wouldn't be too bright for him.

It's funny, because it was a Friday, and I was working at the University of Wisconsin at the time, and they were playing football Saturday against UNLV. I wanted him to wear red. The red onesie we had for him had a baseball on it, not a football. It didn't matter though, so I dressed him in the red onesie and khaki shorts. We fed him then we drove him to the sitter. Erin, my wife, sat in the back and played with him on the way there. She had a little frog thing that played music and lit up. He was playing with that with her.

Like most first-time parents, my wife and I did all the research on day-care centers versus in-home daycare. We decided to go with an in-home daycare provider, somebody that was referred to us from my wife's work. This sitter had watched other children whose parents worked with my wife. Another employee was taking her three-year-old daughter there at the time.

So we thought we had found the perfect spot. He was going to be the only newborn there. The sitter had a five-year-old son who was starting kindergarten. He was not going to be there during the day. The sitter did have a two-year-old daughter, but Lincoln would be the only newborn with this woman. We thought that was good thing, lots of attention.

We dropped Lincoln off that morning. Around noon, Erin called me. She said the sitter had called her and told her that Lincoln had stopped breathing. He wasn't responding and she had called the ambulance. By the time Erin got the call, Lincoln was already on his way to the hospital.

We got to the hospital as quickly as we could. When we got there, we were taken to a small conference room where two physicians met us, one an emergency physician and the other a child abuse pediatrician. They wouldn't let us see Lincoln. They asked us a bunch of questions, how was he in the morning, how was he interacting. We had no idea what was going on. We told them everything about that morning. He had been fine. He was laughing and cooing on the way to the drop off. We kept asking when we could see Lincoln.

I think they told us right then that the little boy we dropped off in the morning wasn't going to be the same little boy we would be taking home, even if we did get to take him home. Something bad had happened. They thought that he might have been abused. We were stunned. We had put our son in that situation. We live with that guilt every day.

The only thing I wish would have happened differently at the hospital is that they would have let us go in and see him first before questioning us. But maybe that's part of the police stuff, maybe they were worried about us seeing him and changing stories or something. That was the hardest part, sitting in that room for probably an hour before we got to see him.

It was tough when we first saw him because he had all those tubes and a machine was breathing for him. I remember seeing his eyes. They were just barely open. I couldn't see his pupils. I thought, "This isn't good" even as I tried to remain positive.

Two detectives came in and interviewed us separately. I went with one detective, Erin the other. The detective who interviewed me had me go through the whole scenario, what happened, what the morning was like. That was really the only time I felt like they were coming after me. I watch TV shows. I know the dad is usually looked at more than anybody else just because statistically he's the most likely perpetrator. It was a good hour that he just kept going back and forth, back and forth about the timeline. What was the morning like? Who fed him? Who dressed him? Who took him out of the car seat? At the end, the detective said to me that if he found out I was lying he was going to come back after me. I told him, "Then I guess I won't hear from you again."

Lincoln was in the hospital for four days before he died. Once we were allowed to be with Lincoln, we never left his side. We were with him 24/7 during those four days. We didn't want to leave him alone.

Whenever a detective or other professional came in to talk to us, I would invite them into Lincoln's room. I wanted them to meet him and see for themselves the devastation that had been done to him.

The doctors did all sorts of tests. In the end, they told us that there was no brain activity. He was never going to come out of it, never going to come home. All that was left was for us to make a decision about was when to turn the machines off, when basically he was going to take his last breath. We were shocked even though we knew this moment could be coming. We had been praying for a miracle. We didn't answer at first. Over the next couple of hours, on two occasions someone came back and asked us if we had made a decision yet. It was the only time I got upset with anyone at the hospital. I told them, "We're not doing this today. We will tell you when." Eventually, we did agree to discontinue life support. At the end, a nurse helped us cut some hair and make hand prints and footprints.

The nurses and the doctors were awesome. We had all of our family there. We were over the limit as far as visitors, but they never made an issue of it. They let us all be there with him. An important thing that everyone needs to realize is that it's not just mom and dad who are going through this: it's grandparents, aunts and uncles, nieces and nephews. Even now, we have the task of trying to explain to our other children what happened and why. I think it's important for everybody to understand that other people are affected as well.

The sitter was arrested three months after Lincoln died. Then there was the court process and sitting through the court proceedings, all the experts and all the testimony. We felt like we were on trial, because the defense was trying to suggest that we had done something wrong. That was all very difficult.

There have been several court appeals since the sitter was convicted. The most recent was the Medill Justice Project trying to get access to some medical records for an appeal. They wanted six photos. The appeal was eventually denied.

Somehow a journalism student from Medill School of Journalism got a hold of our home number and called our home. We've had two children since Lincoln died and we decided my wife would just stay home and raise them. She was home when the call came in. They called out of the blue and totally shocked her, really upset her. She ended up telling them to call back when I was home.

The student told me that there were some new theories about what had happened. I asked her what those theories were. She told me that maybe my wife dropped him when she fell asleep while rocking him that morning, or that I had dropped him when handing him off to the sitter. It was very upsetting to hear a person basically accuse us. It takes quite a bit to get me upset but I was physically shaking on the phone. I just hung up. They never called back. I know that she was only a student, maybe trying to win some award for her school, but this was our life, our child she was talking about. It was very upsetting.

A support group that had seen our son's obituary in the paper reached out to us. They said that they met once a month and if we ever wanted to come and share our story we could. We started doing that. That was really helpful, just to be able to go to talk to people who actually had experienced the loss of a child. Their situations were obviously not the same as ours. They were families who had lost a child in childbirth or from an illness or an accident. It wasn't the same but just talking to people who had gone through loss and who could understand the feelings you had and the guilt that you carry with you, was very helpful. I would say the support groups were key for us and helped us understand what was normal and what wasn't, that really there is no normal. It's just how you respond.

My wife and I lean on each other a lot. I think one of the keys for us was that we had learned pretty early on, it might have been one of the doctors who had told us, that no two people deal with these things the same way. They told us not to judge one another, if one of us was more or less emotional than the other at any given time. My wife handled it one way. I handled it another. I wanted to be around children just to, I don't know, maybe have something to smile about. My wife didn't really want to be around children so much. We obviously handled it differently. I think knowing that was normal helped us.

A really important thing that helps both Erin and I is our faith. We both believe that one day we will see Lincoln again. Having that knowledge and belief was key to us getting through the darkest days.

Another thing that Erin and I have talked about was not letting this change us, not letting it make us negative. This experience has definitely changed our outlook on life, don't get me wrong, but we cherish every moment we have together as a family and don't take any moment for granted.

Our family is very important to us. Our parents, brothers and sisters were all very supportive. My wife went back to work and they were very supportive there. It was difficult for her because the sitter's husband worked at the same office. The office though did a good job of keeping their work spaces separate. He didn't, as far as we know, have anything to do with our son's death, but it was still very difficult for her.

We went to Denver a couple years ago to speak at the National Shaken Baby Conference. That was a great experience and a big challenge for us because we were leaving our children for the first time. I also spoke at a law school. It was helpful just being able to share our experiences, share Lincoln's story, try to keep his memory alive, and not let his name just go into the wind. It will be 10 years in a few days. I think about that, it's kind of crazy that he'd be 10 in two weeks.

My wife and I both run. There is a Thanksgiving Day run called the Berbee Derby. We always put a team together. We call it Lincoln's Road Runners. We invite all sorts of people to join us. Some years we get a good turnout, some years not so good. Every year, we also give out bracelets to the Berbee Derby team and our family with Lincoln's name on them.

I also think it's important to acknowledge the impact this case had on the nurses, doctors, detectives, victim witness advocates, and district attorney staff. Seeing each of them at the trial, seeing their emotions throughout the process, showed us how invested they were in obtaining justice for Lincoln. To this day, we are still in contact with many of the individuals who worked our case.

I will do anything I can to keep Lincoln's memory alive. If I can talk to someone and prevent at least one family from going through this then Lincoln's legacy will live on and something good can come from this.


A common subplot in most, if not all, of the stories in this book is the role of the courts in protecting children, in punishing the guilty, and in protecting the innocent. As important as this role is, one would hope that the courts would always make decisions using the very best science and the most objective measures of fairness. One would hope.

## CHAPTER EIGHT

# The Courtroom: Triumph of Style over Substance

Child abuse pediatricians testify in court on matters of child welfare but not as often as one might think. In my program, where we see 1,200 children a year, I testify at most a dozen times each year.

In Maine, as in other states, there are two court systems, civil and criminal (Myers 1992; St. Onge and Elam 2000). These two systems are not just for child abuse cases but for all court litigation. When dealing with child abuse, the goals and standards of these two systems are quite different.

Civil court, sometimes referred to as family court, is presided over by a judge not a jury. The issue at hand is whether the child was abused, not necessarily by whom. The goal is protection of the child with the applicable laws being the child welfare statutes. The burden of proof is "preponderance of the evidence," sometimes referred to as "more likely than not." Child welfare hearings are not public. In Maine, the plaintiff, child protective services, is represented by the attorney general's office, while the defendants, usually the parent or parents, are represented by private counsel. If the child is found to be in jeopardy of abuse, the final issue to be decided is how to keep the child safe. If a child protective case eventually reaches the point of termination of parental rights, the burden of proof for the state is "clear and convincing evidence," greater than "preponderance," but less than "beyond a reasonable doubt," the standard for criminal conviction.

Criminal court is quite different. The issue at hand is innocence or guilt of a defendant. The trier of fact is a judge or a jury depending on the defendant's choice. The goal is conviction of a perpetrator and the applicable standards are the criminal code. The plaintiff is the state represented by the district attorney's office, or, in the case of a homicide, by the criminal division of the attorney general's office, at least in Maine. Criminal trials take place in public. The burden of proof is "beyond a reasonable doubt."

As with court systems, there are two types of witnesses, material and expert (Stern 1997). A material witness is a witness of fact—someone who describes what they saw or heard. An expert witness offers an opinion about the meaning of what was seen or heard. For example, in the case of a pattern bruise, a material witness would describe the bruising as they saw it. An expert would say what it was a pattern of, such as a belt or hand, and whether the pattern represented inflicted injury or not. According to the federal rules of evidence, if specialized knowledge will help the trier of fact (judge or jury) understand the evidence, a qualified person (the expert) may render an opinion.

What constitutes responsible expert testimony and, more important, what constitutes irresponsible expert testimony has been a significant area of discussion and concern in the field of child abuse (Chadwick 1990; Block 1999). This has not just been an issue for child abuse cases but has long been a concern in all forms of expert testimony.

Many professional organizations have developed standards for responsible expert testimony (Paul and Narang 2017). Standards include current experience and knowledge specific to the area of injury and interpretation of the medical facts based on currently accepted criteria. It is the duty of the expert to act independently of the parties, express only genuinely held opinions, never omit conflicting data, state the basis of the opinion, and acknowledge weaknesses in the opinion. All this is to be desired but does not always happen. Most problematic, the trier of fact is sometimes left to interpret conflicting medical testimony with little educational basis for doing so.

---

**Christine Barron, MD, Providence, Rhode Island**

The very first time I ever testified was in a child welfare hearing. No one had prepared me. In the hearing, the alleged perpetrators were sitting on the other side of the table from me. This was quite disconcerting. Every time I spoke, they glared at me. The defense attorney was also difficult. He kept yelling at me. At one point, I said, "Sorry, can you please repeat the question? Your yelling is distracting me." The attorney was reprimanded for yelling.

I learned so much from that case, particularly about documentation. I had talked to the primary care provider ahead of time and had documented that I had talked to him, but I had not included the details of the discussion in my report. The defense attorney kept hammering at me, "How are we to believe your memory? There's nothing documented anywhere."

About a month after my testimony, while the hearing was still going on, I was contacted by the CPS attorney who asked me if I knew the child protective worker who had investigated the case. I told him I did. He said to me, "Have you ever told him that this child was not abused?" I told him, "Absolutely not." He said, "Well, I need you to come back. The worker just perjured himself during his testimony."

I went back and was asked if I knew this person. I said, "Yes." I was asked "Have you ever had a conversation with him?" I said "Yes." I was asked "Have you ever told him this child was not abused?" I said "No." The defense attorney got up and said, "How are we to believe you, Dr. Barron?" I said, "Because I have never said to anyone at any time that this child was not abused." The worker subsequently lost his job.

This experience was really eye-opening for me. The case involved a teenage girl who was sexually abused by her adoptive father. This social worker, who had lied on the stand, had worked with the family through the adoption. When this girl disclosed abuse, he said to her, "I know these parents. They are so nice. There's no way that they've done this to you."

I never would have thought a professional would do that. I was just shocked. I couldn't believe a professional would try to influence a victim into saying that something had not happened when it had and then lie under oath. I learned so much from that experience, particularly about documentation.

### Amanda Brownell, MD, Cincinnati, Ohio

I enjoy the challenge of court. It's one of the reasons I chose child abuse as a profession. You don't really know what to expect. I think it is interesting to watch the jury's reaction to the testimony. It is also a challenge to get your technical medical points across to a lay person.

In one of my earliest cases, I was allowed to watch the proceedings after I testified. The defense attorney said to the judge, "We just heard from some woman who works with children all day." I was flabbergasted! I know that it was just a tactic to discredit me, but it was a more personal attack than I had previously experienced. "Just some woman," indeed! The judge said to him, "Well, she is a physician. She is an expert witness. She is not a faith healer. She is not a witch doctor."

I was disappointed by the defense tactic but impressed with the judge.

**Alex V. Levin, MD, MHSc, Philadelphia, Pennsylvania**

Golf is the most frustrating sport on the planet for me. It's the only sport where no matter how much I play, I still don't get any better (and sometimes I get worse!). In order to keep playing I had to come to the realization that the joy of the game was being outdoors and solving the challenges of the course, not winning. It should be fun.

Court is the same way. Court is not about the truth. Court is not about an accurate medical diagnosis. If I can accept that and just think of myself as an objective educator for the judge and jury, then I can enjoy it. I try to divorce myself from the outcome, because I have no stake in the outcome. I don't know who is guilty or not. I can only speak to what happened to the child based on the medical facts of the case.

My job is to be a teacher. I love to teach. That's easy for me. All the craziness that goes on with attorneys and opposing medical witnesses is sad. It's frustrating. But I appreciate the overwhelming burden of the jury and the judge. They don't understand much of the medical evidence. My job is to try and make that evidence clear and understandable.

I do believe in the adversarial system. As much as there is intellectual dishonesty in the courtroom, it is still important to realize that such testimony keeps us honest. It keeps us asking questions. In this field, we need to be sure we're right, because the stakes are not just medical, they're legal. People do go to jail. We don't put people in jail, the courts do. But, we inform the courts about the medical diagnosis which may implicate abuse as the mechanism of injury.

The court has to decide who the perpetrator may be. I think these crazy theories of vaccines and other things challenge us to do good research. I've certainly done research to make sure our thinking is medically and scientifically correct in direct response to legal challenges.

**Kent P. Hymel, MD, Hershey, Pennsylvania**

I no longer try to be the answer to everyone's needs in our field. I don't put myself out there any more as an expert who testifies against child abuse denialists (those who would argue that abusive head trauma does not exist, for example). It was burning me out. The novel, unsupported theories being thrown out in court took so much preparation to debunk that most of what I was doing was rereading the same papers over and over just to keep them fresh in my mind.

It was also keeping me from achieving my main goal which is development of a screening tool for abusive head trauma. I want to focus on something that will leave the field better than I found it. Contentious opposing testimony was interfering with that, so I just stopped.

I do have very memorable court cases. In one case, I spoke to the parents of a severely head-injured child. I told them that I'd done all of the tests I could think of to evaluate the possibility of conditions other than trauma, but that I could find nothing else. I told them that I concluded that their child's condition was caused by trauma and that, in the absence of an accidental explanation, I concluded that he had been abused. I told them that I recognized how difficult this was for them to hear, but that I would explain everything. I would answer all their questions. I would try to support them through this trying process. I told the father that I wanted him to understand that, because his son had become symptomatic in his care, the police were going to be focusing their attention on him.

The father didn't say much. The mother was in shock. They went home that evening. The next morning only the mother came back. She told me that as they were driving home, her husband pulled the car over and said, "I can't continue to lie to you. I need to tell you what I did to our son because, if I don't, he may lose both of us and that would be horrible. You should not be taken out of his life. I'm going to take you home and then I'm going to go to the police and tell them exactly what I did." I really admired that profound moment of courage. It resonated with me for a long time. I think about that father quite frequently.

I had another case, similar but with a different outcome. I told the parents that I believed their child had been abused and that it happened while their baby was in the care of the father. I told them, "If you have additional information, if there's some other explanation that you haven't yet told me, please don't take too much longer to share it because, if child protective services doesn't know who to protect your child from, they may have to elect to protect your child from both of you."

Neither one said anything, but as I left, the father followed me out and said, "Can I talk to you for a few minutes?" I said, "Sure." He said, "How sure are you?" I said, "I feel pretty confident in my diagnosis." He asked, "So what do you think is going to happen?" I said, "Honestly, I think that your child will be taken from you. I think that the authorities will be convinced these injuries happened while your child was in your care, and I think there's a good possibility that you will be arrested." He said, "What will happen if I'm arrested?" I said, "There will come a time, maybe nine, ten months from now, when I'll walk into a courtroom and raise my right hand. You'll be sitting at the defense table and you and I will look at each other and we'll both remember that I told you this moment would come." I added, "I hope it doesn't come to that. If you have something to say, please say it now, ask for help, acknowledge that you need help, so that it doesn't come to that, because then it'll be too late." Tears streamed down his face. He started to say something but then he stopped himself and said, "I just can't." He turned around and walked back in the room. Sure enough, 10 months later, I raised my right hand in the courtroom. The father and I stared at each other. I have no doubt that we both were remembering our previous conversation.

In the first case, a father found the courage to acknowledge what he did. In the second case, a father came close but couldn't quite do it.

It's a privilege and a responsibility to be part of these deeply personal moments in the lives of families. I think this profession calls on us to hold that responsibility as a solemn duty.

### Emalee G. Flaherty, MD, Chicago, Illinois

I have to say that court was always painful for me. I haven't had to testify since I retired but I have a case coming up now. I really dread having to go back and relearn all the science.

I hate all those physicians testifying in areas they have no expertise in. A doctor from my area started testifying for the defense. He has said things in court like "rib fractures can be from normal handling." There is no evidence in the literature to support that opinion.

Since he started testifying, the prosecutors have been reluctant to take a case to trial he is scheduled to testify in and possibly lose.

In one case in which he testified, the child was returned to his parents and came back later severely injured. The point is not who wins or loses in court. Children are unprotected because of this kind of testimony.

### Lynn K. Sheets, MD, Milwaukee, Wisconsin

A case that really had an impact on me involved deaf parents. Their infant son came into the hospital with severe inflicted head trauma. I interviewed each parents separately. This ended up being one of only a handful of cases in my career when a parent, in this case the father, confessed to me.

I remember very clearly talking with him. We were in the emergency room using a signing interpreter. I don't confront parents even when I don't believe their story. In this case, I simply asked him to explain to me what had happened. I told him I was trying to understand what he was telling me. After a while, he signed that he wanted to tell me what really happened.

He told me the baby was crying, crying, crying. He couldn't get the baby to stop. He kept trying to move his son's face away, so he wouldn't see the crying. The baby had neck bruising from where he pushed his head to one side. Then, in exasperation, he shook him and threw him into the crib. As soon as he did that, the baby stopped crying.

I asked him how he knew the baby was crying since he couldn't hear. He looked at me incredulously and signed, "I knew he was crying. I could see he was crying." Then he told me how inadequate he felt, not being able to get his son to stop crying.

I was overwhelmed with empathy for him. The confession seemed to me to be heartfelt. Of course, he went to jail. He lost his son and his wife. I've thought about that father so many times.

I struggle thinking about that remorseful father, that ruined family, and that brain-damaged baby boy growing up without his father. There's something that doesn't seem right about that. If you have a father who's done something really awful, but is remorseful, there has to be safety first of course, but couldn't there be some sort of consequence that takes into account remorse, something that involves punishment but also a chance at reunification?

### Sandeep K. Narang, MD, JD, Chicago, Illinois

Before becoming a child abuse pediatrician, I was a prosecuting attorney for the Navy. I was assigned a difficult case involving a 10-year-old girl who had been sexually abused by her military stepfather. I was an inexperienced prosecutor fumbling my way through the case. The military has what is known as an Article 32 hearing, sort of equivalent to a grand jury. I hadn't thought through the circumstances of her having to testify at the Article 32 hearing. I had thought she would testify in a large conference room with sufficient distance between her and her stepfather. But the room ended up being very small and she had to sit no more than a foot away from him. I still wonder if I did her more harm than good.

Her strength astounded me. She turned her face so she could not see him, and then, in a clear voice, proceeded to tell the Article 32 officer exactly what he had done to her. Because of her strong testimony, her stepfather pled guilty.

After that I realized that I needed to do a better job. I had already decided to go to medical school but this case confirmed for me that I wanted to go into pediatrics and then child abuse pediatrics. I wanted to help abused children.

In many ways, I found the military court system particularly well suited to handle expert testimony. I find the civilian system much less adept. In the latter, judges and juries are generally unskilled at understanding and interpreting expert testimony. Military juries are well educated, thoughtful, and attentive. I usually felt that their verdicts were correct, even if unfavorable to the side I represented.

It is particularly interesting that military jurors can ask questions of a witness after first having their questions screened by a judge. I would often find that their questions were better than some of mine.

In the U.S. civilian system, all sorts of crazy, unfiltered expert opinion can be presented. Judges and juries are ill equipped to judge the validity of the testimony. One change that might help would be to have judges receive scientific training.

### Stephen C. Boos, MD, Springfield, Massachusetts

When I was in the military, I was asked to be a child abuse consultant for the defense. This is something that happens in the military. The defense team is assigned a doctor who helps them understand the medical aspects of the case.

The case was about sexual abuse. The prosecution was based, in part, on a disclosure that happened in therapy. The young girl didn't really want to go to therapy. The therapist testified in court that she said to the child, "Look, you can tell me about what your dad did to you and then maybe you won't have to come here anymore, or you can continue to deny that anything happened to you and then you're going to have to keep coming here every week." After that, the child gave a very minimal disclosure of fondling. This felt to me like a coerced disclosure.

For me though, the major problem with the prosecution was the doctor they called as their medical expert. He described mounds (bumps) on the edge of the hymen as evidence of sexual abuse. This was at a point in the evolution of the medical science of diagnosing sexual abuse where study after study had found that mounds on the edge of the hymen were normal and not signs of abuse.

This doctor did take pictures, but they were so bad, they were uninterpretable. In court, he not only said that the mounds were diagnostic of sexual abuse, but that the girl had disclosed to him during the exam, a disclosure that he did not document in his medical record.

Rather than continue as a behind-the-scenes consultant, I ended up testifying for the defense. I testified that mounds were not a sign of abuse and that I saw no medical evidence to conclude that this child had been sexually abused.

The prosecution asked me if I thought the other doctor was incompetent. I thought for a while then answered that he was incompetent in the opinion he rendered on the witness stand. I said that he clearly did not know the status of the current medical literature on sexual abuse. I did say that I could not comment on his competence beyond this case, but that I thought his testimony was indeed incompetent.

I thought I had testified appropriately but on reflection I was concerned that in the transition from consultant to witness I had emotionally joined with the defense team. I think that I adhered to appropriate professional limits but by the same token, I think I was in a very dangerous emotional position, because I had joined the defense team.

### Suzanne P. Starling, MD, San Diego, California

Two legal cases stand out in my mind. Both cases involved parents who had been accused of abuse of their young children. In the first case, I was asked by a defense attorney and in the second by a prosecutor to review the medical records.

In the first case, the parents had lost custody of their surviving twin after one twin died from abusive head trauma. When I reviewed the materials for the defense attorney, it was clear to me that the children's babysitter, not the parents, had been responsible for the death of the child.

As a result of my review, the parents were able to get their surviving child back and there later was a successful prosecution of the babysitter. The baby's parents came to the Shaken Baby Conference in Salt Lake City and gave me a bouquet of roses with a balloon and a teddy bear. They cried and hugged me. They told me. "You saved our lives. Thank you so much." It was just amazing. The teddy bear still sits on my bookshelf at work. When I first started out in this field I thought what many people still think, that I would only be testifying against parents not for them. It was very gratifying to help that family.

In the second case, I was asked by a prosecutor to be a witness in a child homicide case, even though I had not personally evaluated the child. A mother had been charged with shaking her son to death. I was told she had confessed, but as I reviewed her confession, I realized that what she had confessed to was knocking him off a tricycle 10 days before his death. The detective had said to her, "So, you're saying you knocked him off the tricycle. If we told you that knocking him off that tricycle is what killed him, would you say that you killed him?" She said, "If that's what killed him, then yeah, I killed him".

After they interviewed the mother, the police stopped any further investigation. They never interviewed other caregivers of the child. They just charged her with the crime. I told the prosecutor that knocking him off his tricycle 10 days before he died could not have resulted in the injuries that killed the child. She hadn't even been home when her son died. The district attorney dropped the charges against her and the police reopened the investigation.

We can make a difference not only by helping children but by helping families as well. Because of these two cases, I have focused some of my research on accidental injuries that can be confused with abuse. Many people don't understand that we have as much of a vested interest in protecting families as we do in protecting children.

## About Jasmine

I don't remember Jasmine very well. I do remember the trial. It was my first time testifying, my first time ever in a courtroom.

I was in my last year of my second residency, this one in emergency medicine. A nine-year-old girl had come to the emergency room saying that she had been sexually abused by her father. I thought her examination was normal but, looking back after 30 years of child abuse practice, I doubt I had any idea what I was looking for. This was 1980. The world literature on what to look for when examining a sexually abused child consisted of only a few published articles.

When the case went to trial, I was surprised to be called to testify by the defense. The father's attorney led me into a small conference room and read the questions he was going to ask me in court. I was grateful for the opportunity to go over my testimony in advance, despite my misgiving that I was testifying for the defense.

The courtroom was small and crowded—judge, 12 jurors, defense and prosecution attorneys, and several observers in pew-like seats in the back. I sat nervously on the witness stand to the judge's left, desperately trying to orient myself to this strange environment.

The animated defense attorney, often smiling knowingly to the jury, asked me to describe in great detail the child's normal examination. He even had me draw on a blackboard. The judge and jury listened intently. The prosecutor looked like he was falling asleep. The jury, I am sure, was left believing that the normal examination meant this girl had not been abused, that she had in fact lied about being abused by her father.

If I had been asked what a normal examination meant, I would have said that a normal examination meant nothing. For any number of reasons, most children who are sexually abused have a normal examination. The old axiom still holds true, "Absence of evidence is not evidence of absence." But I wasn't asked about any of that, not even in cross-examination by the bored prosecutor who should have known better.

After my testimony, just before stepping off the stand, I turned to the judge and asked him if I could say something. I wanted desperately to tell the jury that they should ignore the normal examination and that they should just listen to the child. The startled judge looked at me as if I was out of my mind and firmly told me that I was only allowed to speak in response to a question.

Chastised and embarrassed, I left the courtroom, certain that my unskilled testimony would mean a sex offender would go free, that a sexually abused child would continue to be at risk. My only consolation from that day was what I learned. I learned about the importance of pre-trial preparation, about how to conduct myself on the witness stand, about how to make sure that what I needed to say was said, and most important, about how the courtroom can sometimes be a forum for style over substance.

## About Ricky

Since that first somewhat disillusioning experience, I have testified many times. My first high-profile cases also happened to be the first and only time a Maine criminal case was broadcasted on court TV. The following factual information is taken from that broadcast recording.

Ricky, a four-year-old boy, died after his foster mother pushed him and he fell to the floor in his bedroom. At his autopsy, Ricky had bleeding on his brain and extensive injuries to his skin. The cause of death was listed as aspiration of vomit following a concussion.

Normally, I do not get involved in cases when a child dies outside the hospital. These cases typically go directly to the state medical examiner. In this case, however, I was asked by the prosecuting attorney and the medical examiner to offer an opinion as a child abuse specialist about the cause or causes of Ricky's skin injuries.

I read the reports and studied the photographs. I didn't count the skin injuries, but everyone, prosecution and defense alike, agreed that there were 127. Many of these were deep, raking fingernail scratches involving the back of Ricky's ears, his buttocks, and the underside of his scrotum. There was also bruising of the buttocks in a pattern that could only have been caused by spanking. Finally, and perhaps most significantly, there was a large bruise and significant swelling of the right side of Ricky's face and ear. It was my opinion that this child had been profoundly physically abused. The skin injuries were undeniably inflicted.

But as I looked more closely at the records, as I saw the evidence of swelling and bruising of the face, as I saw evidence of direct brain trauma, I felt that not only had Ricky been beaten savagely, but I agreed with the prosecutor that "Ricky had been disciplined to death."

When I met with the prosecutor to discuss my testimony, it quickly became apparent to me that the medical examiner and I differed in our respective opinions about the cause of Ricky's death. The medical examiner felt that Ricky had died from the unintended consequence of a simple fall. He had been knocked unconscious from the fall and suffocated on his own vomit. I felt that inflicted trauma, not the fall, had caused the head injuries that ultimately led to Ricky's death.

Whether I was correct or not, this was not good. In medicine, as in most fields, professional relationships are critically important. In this case, our diverging opinions, played out on court TV, ultimately harmed my relationship with the medical examiner's office for many years. During those years, I often wondered if offering an opinion about the cause of Ricky's death had been worth the loss of collegial trust.

At the trial, the prosecutor's argument was simple. Ricky had been "disciplined to death." His foster mother had repeatedly slapped his face, spanked his bottom, raked her fingernails across his buttocks and scrotum, as she yanked his clothing off, all because Ricky had enraged her by "intentionally" peeing on her floor. It was the blows to his face and head, not the fall the prosecutor said, that had killed him.

The defense argument was more convoluted. After she pushed him into his room, where he fell and lost consciousness, his foster mother took him into the bathroom. She splashed water on his face. She slapped his face. She tried to give him mouth-to-mouth resuscitation. He vomited. She denied raking her fingernails over his buttocks and scrotum. She denied hitting him except to resuscitate him. This was all an unfortunate accident in a child who had caused many of the injuries to himself.

It is odd watching the court TV video now. I find my palms getting damp and my heart racing almost as if I were in that courtroom again. There was a large audience. There were TV cameras and bright lights. I was testifying against the state medical examiner. The visceral memory remains even now after 20 years.

It is odd also listening again to the testimony of the defense experts. One speculated that Ricky's swollen brain was due to increased levels of carbon dioxide, a novel and scientifically unsupported theory. Another speculated that this child with no preexisting medical condition had a seizure and that the seizure had led to vomiting, aspiration, and death. Another speculated that many of the injuries on Ricky's body were self-inflicted because he suffered from an attachment disorder, this in a child with no history of self-injury. Another expert, who never saw the autopsy photographs of Ricky's injuries, speculated that a fall from a standing height onto a carpeted floor could have caused the massive facial bruising. Another speculated that some of the clearly inflicted adult fingernail injuries were from his foster mother's jewelry. I wonder what would have been found if a forensics lab had tested her nails.

At trial, Ricky's foster mother admitted that one of her techniques for trying to manage the behavior of this attachment disordered child was to further traumatize him by isolating him from the rest of the family. She also spanked him, even going so far as to use a wooden spoon. Physical discipline is a violation of the regulations governing foster care.

According to his foster mother, on the day of his death, Ricky "intentionally" urinated on the floor six times. After the first time, she spanked him and put rubber pants on him. She told him that, if he was going to act like a baby, she was going to treat him like one. After Ricky urinated the sixth time, she got "really angry" and spanked him again. She then told him that she had had enough of him for that day, took him by the scruff of the neck, and pushed him into his room where he fell. He never got up.

At one point during her testimony, she said she had vowed to herself, after an earlier spanking, never to hit Ricky again, because doing so hurt her more than it hurt him. This was a profoundly narcissistic statement. She could not see how these spankings hurt Ricky, only how they affected her. Tellingly, when being asked by her own attorney how she felt when Ricky fell to the ground, she replied, "My whole world had turned upside down"—this while Ricky lay dying.

In the end, the judge did not find the evidence sufficient to convict her of manslaughter. How could he when faced with contradictory testimony from so many professionals? The judge felt that the fall could have caused the concussion and that the concussion had the unintended consequence of causing Ricky's death. I would agree with the judge's opinion on this, not about the truth of it, but about the sufficiency of the evidence given the conflicting testimony. The judge also did not find her guilty of aggravated assault, an opinion I did not agree with given the multitude of injuries Ricky had endured. The judge did find her guilty of assault, specifically of spanking Ricky and raking his genitals and buttocks with her fingernails. He also found not a shred of evidence that Ricky self-mutilated. He sentenced her to one year in prison.

The case was headline news in Maine during the trial. Not only experts but communities took sides. The foster mother's church and a local school raised money for her and her family. A local pastor said that he believed nothing bad had happened in that home. I wonder what the pastor would have said had he seen the autopsy photographs.

I used to believe that any parent could abuse a child given the right risk factors and triggers. But most parents never abuse their children. Few parents kill a child and even fewer of these are the child's mother. Even rarer is the perpetrator a foster mother.

As far as is known, there have been two children who were abused and died in the care of a foster mother in Maine. The first was Ricky. The second was Logan.

Five-year-old Logan was removed from the custody of her mother and placed in foster care. In the foster home, Logan was reported to have meltdowns and uncontrollable screaming. Her foster mother, unable to control Logan's behavior, used progressively harsher discipline techniques, even covering Logan with a blanket and lying on top of her while bargaining with her for the release of one limb at a time.

One day, Logan so infuriated her foster mother that she placed her in a highchair in the basement and wrapped her in 42 feet of duct tape. She wrapped the duct tape under Logan's chin, over her head, and across her mouth. Logan suffocated to death.

The foster mother was convicted of manslaughter and sentenced to 20 years in prison. The court found that the relationship between Logan and her foster mother had become a test of wills that the foster mother was determined to win. The foster mother could not accept that a five-year-old girl might get the best of her. Despite all her training, experience, knowledge, and her awareness of the rules and regulations for a foster parent, she mummified Logan and left her to struggle and die alone.

Ricky's and Logan's deaths, because they were wards of the state, raised important questions about the child welfare system, who should be in foster care, how well trained should foster parent be, and how closely children should be monitored by their state workers. But in the very appropriate rush to study the child welfare system in these cases, a more fundamental question was never asked. Are there characteristics in a foster parent, indeed in any seemingly educated parent, which might signal a problem? I believe there are.

I have always been struck by the similarities between Ricky's and Logan's foster mothers. Both were highly educated. Both had training in child development. Both found the foster children difficult, if not impossible, to manage. Neither sought out professional help for their child management difficulties. Neither was well supervised by the child welfare system. When faced with a defiant child, both reverted to primitive discipline techniques.

Of the many lessons of Logan and Ricky's deaths, one of the most important ones, I believe, is the grave danger, the life-threatening danger, of placing a child with the wrong caretaker. Of course, the first lesson is to be absolutely certain that foster care is the right answer to begin with.

The deaths of these two children are not typical of most child abuse deaths. Most child abuse deaths are perpetrated by parents or partners of parents, not by foster parents. During the 10 years between Ricky's and Logan's deaths, 20 children were killed in their own homes in Maine by a parent or parent's partner.

Since Logan's death, Maine has taken steps to decrease the number of children needing foster care through more intensive family preservation efforts and, when placement outside the home cannot be avoided, using kinship placement, if available.

Attention must be paid to every child who dies. Lessons must be learned from every death. One of the lessons to be learned from the death of these two children is how horribly things can go wrong for children when care is not taken to ensure the best placement, how horribly things can go wrong when the system whose job it is to ensure safety fails in its duty.

Child abuse work is stressful. How can it not be? It's not that there is stress but how that stress is handled that is important. It can be handled in a healthy way leading to growth or in an unhealthy way, leading to burnout, or worse, loss of objectivity.

## CHAPTER NINE

# Vicarious Trauma: "How Can You Do This Work?"

## About Angel

Angel was then and is, even now months later, one of the most beautiful babies I have ever seen, and I have seen many in my 30 years as a child abuse pediatrician. To look at her, asleep against her adoptive mother's shoulder, one could never have guessed the damage she had suffered.

I first met then three-months-old Angel on Christmas Eve in the pediatric intensive care unit. She had been admitted the evening before in a coma. Her father told the hospital staff that he had picked her up from her crib to change her soaked diaper and, as he did so, she slipped from his grasp and fell back into her crib. He said she went limp and stopped breathing. He rushed her to his car and drove wildly to the hospital. Efforts to resuscitate her were successful but the damage had already been done.

I was called in to see her after a CT scan of her head showed subdural hematomas (bleeding on the surface of the brain from trauma). Later, an MRI found evidence of extensive brain injury. An examination of her eyes by an ophthalmologist found severe retinal hemorrhages (bleeding in the back of the eyes from trauma).

Angel's mother was at work when the injury occurred. She told me, what her boyfriend had told her, that Angel had fallen from his grasp into the crib. She said she had no reason to doubt his explanation, but, looking back, I think she did.

Angel's father told me that the baby had "peed everywhere," on her clothes and in her bed. When he picked her up, she slipped from his grasp and fell onto the mattress. She immediately lost consciousness.

He acted nervous and was vague in his answers. When I probed for more information, he exploded and asked me why I didn't believe him. I told him I was just trying to figure out how a fall like that could cause such severe trauma. But he told me nothing more, so I ended the interview.

Later, Angel's mother came up to me and said that she now knew what really had happened to Angel. After he talked to me, her boyfriend confessed to her that he had shaken Angel. She told me that he wanted to talk to me.

I went into Angel's room. Her father was sitting on a cot with his head in his hands, Angel's mother sat by his side, consoling him. He didn't look like a bad person, perpetrators rarely do.

Before I could speak, he offered, "I'm sorry Doc. I lied. I shook her."

I asked him why he had shaken her. He said, "I picked her up from the crib. She was screaming and kicking and scratching at me and I just lost it. I shook her."

I asked, "Did the fall happen?"

"No Doc. She didn't fall. I shook her."

Finally, "What happened after you shook her?"

"She went limp and stopped breathing. She looked dead. I know what I did was wrong. I'm sorry Doc."

So there it was. I thanked him for telling me the truth. I told him it was the right thing to do.

A year later, Angel's father pled guilty to assault. At his sentencing, he said that he had shaken Angel and that he was sorry. He was sentenced to several years in prison.

But, in the hospital on that Christmas Eve day, all of this had yet to pass. Here was Angel in the ICU, profoundly brain damaged, never to awake, a victim of devastating violence. For all the world, she looked like a beautiful, healthy three-month-old girl about to experience her first Christmas.

I have seen many shaken babies, many victims of abusive head trauma. Yet, it always astounds me how normal many of these babies look, few if any bruises, no obvious fractures, nothing to suggest the abuse they had suffered. To look at Angel in her hospital bed surrounded by beeping instruments and tubes, not responding, a ventilator breathing for her, she looked fine, cherubic.

I saw her one last time several months later. She was accompanied by her adoptive parents. Her functioning at a year was that of a one-month-old.

Her existence, like that of a light switch, was without nuance, flipping between screaming/arching and deep sedation. She was quadriplegic, blind and deaf. Her newly adoptive parents attend to her all day and all night, ceaselessly, religiously. I am not religious myself and had never said to anyone, "May God bless you." I did to them. My eyes filling, I told them they were saints who deserved a special place in heaven.

There is something of a "debate" within the legal community and on the fringes of the medical community about the existence of shaken baby syndrome. One argument offered is that confessions are always coerced. Another is that shaking cannot cause these injuries. Those who would say such things should talk to Angel's father.

But for Angel, none of this matters. Words and events orbit around her like so many errant planets: shaken baby prevention, child protective custody, termination of parental rights, grand jury, criminal prosecution, plea bargain, prison. Unknown and unknowing, immutably beautiful, she spins silently within her own dying sun.


Professionals who work with victims of child abuse may themselves experience psychological trauma from the work. For some, the psychological effects are so painful and disruptive that they simply cannot continue to do the work. For others, although they can continue to do the work, the residual effects can influence their decision making and even influence their day-to-day lives. One term for such effects is "vicarious trauma." Other, often used, terms include "burnout," "counter-transference," "compassion fatigue," "secondary victimization," "secondary traumatic stress disorder," and "critical incident stress" (McCann and Pearlman 1990; Schetky and Devoe 1992).

Counter-transference refers to the psychological reaction a professional has to a patient or situation based on the professional's own previous experiences. Some professionals may overly identify with a victim or even with an alleged perpetrator. Child custody conflicts may stir up unresolved issues with one's own parents. The courtroom is a minefield of counter-transference. It is far too easy on the witness stand to want to please the attorney who called the professional to testify.

Once, as I was finishing my testimony on a sexual abuse case, the prosecutor asked me one final question: "Doctor Ricci, has this child been sexually abused?" I knew the prosecutor wanted me to simply say "yes." But I didn't feel comfortable saying that. I was there to offer an opinion about the injury I saw, not about the ultimate issue of abuse.

Instead of answering the question directly, I spent some time describing the genital injury and how that injury was consistent with penetrating trauma.

I am not sure the jury heard or even understood much of my answer. Afterward, the prosecutor said to me, "I just wanted you to say 'yes'."

The underlying premise of vicarious trauma is that we construct our own sense of reality as we interpret events in our lives. Forged by our experiences, each of us develop our own unique sense of safety in a dangerous world, of trust in others, of power to control our destiny, and of the ability to be intimate. Vicarious trauma tells us that our sense of reality will, of necessity, be altered by the work we do. Thus, safety may turn into irrational fear of assault, trust in others might turn into lack of trust in, for example, babysitters, power to control our own destiny might turn into a sense of abject powerlessness, and ability to be intimate might turn into alienation from friends and colleagues. Symptoms of vicarious trauma may include intrusive imagery, nightmares, emotional numbing, fear, paranoid, depression, and anger. From a work-related perspective the most dangerous symptom is loss of objectivity.

Whether the effects of vicarious trauma are destructive or constructive depends on the extent a professional is able to integrate and transform these experiences into personal and professional insight. In the end, not only our lives but our work teaches us who we are.

In my practice, my professional colleagues—medical, social work, and psychology—meet weekly to talk about the stress of the work. We meet at other times to discuss clinical decision making. These meetings, however, which we call peer supervision, are to talk about our feelings in a safe and supportive environment. We talk to help us gain perspective. We talk so that these feelings do not interfere with our clinical decision making. We talk to purge the harsh demons of our work.

---

**Rachel Berger, MD, MPH, Pittsburgh, Pennsylvania**

I am very good at separating my work life from my home life. I do work at home but mostly on my research. I rarely talk about or think about cases when I am home. I know that it is time for an intervention when I find myself thinking about patients at home.

We are exposed to so much family chaos at work. I need stability in the rest of my life in order to keep doing what I'm doing. I try very hard to put my family first. I have an incredibly supportive husband and family. I think everybody who's in this field has to have at least one person in their life who understands why we do what we do.

My view of the world is completely different now than it would have been if I didn't do this work. Life can be unfair. You get one childhood and many children in our country don't even get that.

There's no question the work changed the kind of parent I am. When one of my children was a freshman in high school, he called me because his class was going to a rally to encourage people to get out and vote. He asked me, "Can my teacher drive me in his car instead of my taking the public bus?" I said, "Is the teacher driving all the other children?" He said, "I don't know." I said, "You need to ask. If the teacher's driving everybody in his car, then yes, you can go. If the teacher's driving only you in his car, then the answer is no." He seemed surprised, "What are you talking about?" I said, "I don't know this teacher." He said, "But he's such a great guy." I told him, "I don't know this teacher. You cannot drive alone with him in the car." He said, "You are totally skewed by your work. You can't even see that people are good." I told him "No, no, no, you don't understand. I know what people are really like."

As I thought about that conversation, I realized that what he was saying to me was that my whole life had been affected by what I do for work. I see people who look like you or me on the outside, yet who are so evil on the inside. I almost wish I didn't know that.

Maybe that's why so many people leave this field. It changes your view of people. If you let it though, it can show you the opposite as well. It can show you the good in people, for example, how some people come forward to take care of children they don't even know.

We also see the resiliency of children. It is incredibly satisfying for me to see a child who was close to death, now thriving. Those kinds of cases carry me through the dark times.

### Christine Barron, MD, Providence, Rhode Island

The work is rewarding for me, particularly when I know I've made a difference in a child's life. I have been fortunate having colleagues who I can talk to about difficult experiences. We have debriefing sessions. A child psychiatrist and a pediatric social worker join us and help facilitate the conversation. I've learned a lot from these meetings, particularly about how to process difficult cases, how to recognize when something is bothering me, and how important it is to talk about what is bothering me about a case.

One of the hardest cases I've seen involved an autistic child who had bruises. Both he and his brother said their mother's boyfriend was hitting them. He had lots of bruises but nothing specific for abuse other than the fact that there were so many of them. CPS and I made a safety plan with his mother. I told her, "CPS and I are making this safety plan with you. Your boyfriend cannot be around your children. If that happens, your children will not return home with you."

I didn't entirely trust this mother so I scheduled a follow-up visit. A week before the scheduled visit, the boys came back. The autistic boy had so many bruises that I had to use a video camera to record them all. The still camera would not have been able to record all of the injuries. Of course the video camera recorded audio as well.

Later, I watched the video so I could accurately document all of his injuries in my written report. The audio was playing in the background. I realized I was being traumatized by the audio. The boy kept saying the boyfriend's name then adding "punish me." He said it over and over again. I finally had to turn off the audio so I could finish my report. I could not listen anymore.

I have a picture of this boy singing and playing Mr. Potato Head with me. It was adorable. He'd gone through a horrible experience, one which I wish I had not allowed him to experience, but here he was playing Mr. Potato Head with me. He's since been adopted by his grandparents and is now thriving. It helps me when I see such a positive outcome from such a horrible situation. I think about that boy all the time.

We have the ability to place children into custody where I work. Because of that, we wield an enormous amount of power. I take it very seriously. It does provide me the opportunity to ensure the safety of a child.

It is difficult though when I see an abused child from a neighboring state. CPS might say to me, "But this is such a nice family." I say to them, "I'm so glad they're a nice family, but this child was abused." Even then, CPS might not listen to me. If the case happened in Rhode Island, I would be able to place the child in a safe environment. A lot of our colleagues would shy away from making these kinds of decisions. It's easier to say, "I'm just giving CPS this information and they will make the decision."

At the end of the day though, I just want to do what is safe for the child. In some abuse cases, I recommend the child stay with their family with a safety plan in place. In other cases, when there is imminent risk of additional injury, I recommend the child be removed from the family.

I have been involved in several cases where the family and even their medical providers do not believe the diagnosis of abuse. In a few cases, doctors have yelled at me because they felt that the families were wonderful. On two occasions, doctors have asked me how I could sleep at night! In one of these cases, I diagnosed abuse and in the other I diagnosed an accidental injury.

I have had families come back after they have finally accepted the diagnosis of abuse and thank me for saving their child's life by placing them into custody. I have testified for the defense about accidental injuries so children would not go into custody or, if they had already been removed, see that they are returned home. I'm fortunate to have a nice balance in my work, to see abuse, but also to see cases that are not abuse, where my opinion keeps a child from unnecessarily being removed for a family.

### Carole Jenny, MD, MBA, Seattle, Washington

I once read a book about sin eaters. A long time ago in Ireland, when a person died, there would be a wake. All the neighbors would bring a sumptuous feast and lay it out on a table. Certain people in the community were designated as sin eaters. They were the only ones who consumed the feast. The idea was that, by doing so, they were consuming all the sins of the dead, so that the dead could go to heaven. In some ways, I think we are sin eaters. We absorb all this tragedy and sadness so that others can be saved.

Every several months I crash. I crashed last week. I had the most horrific sexual abuse case. These beautiful children in a lovely family were sexually abused for years by a predatory relative. It was so sad. The girls were delightful. The day after seeing the girls I called in sick. I stayed in bed with the covers over my head most of the day. In the afternoon, my husband got me out of bed, marched me into the bathroom and said, "Take a shower, go back to work." By the time I got to work, I was fine.

I have two lives. I have my work life and my life life. My work life is all the stressful and painful stuff I see. I see children who die. I see little girls who have been violated. I see terrible things. But then I go home and my life life is my garden, my husband, my children, my grandchildren, and my hobbies. I never read a book where somebody gets murdered or raped. I never go to a movie where people get blown up. I've not seen *Star Wars*, for instance. I flood myself with positive things like classical music, great books, and my wonderful family. I think that's what's kept me going all this time.

### Amanda Brownell, MD, Cincinnati, Ohio

We see children who die from abuse. Often there are other children in the home in need of protection. The way I think about these horrible deaths is that the death of one child may save all the other children in the family from further abuse and possibly even death.

I think having others to talk to, to bounce ideas off of, is helpful as well. We have debriefing sessions after particularly difficult cases. Sometimes we have a chaplain present. But I think the informal sessions are better. It's harder to be open, to say what you are feeling, in front of people you don't know very well.

I also moonlight in an urgent care center. I find it helpful to see loving, non-abusive families. For example, I can have the instant gratification of giving antibiotics to a child for their ear infection. I say to myself, "I can fix this problem and the family leaves happy." It reminds me of why I went into pediatrics in the first place, to see sick babies and make them better. Unfortunately, we can't always do that in our field.

### Allison M. Jackson, MD, MPH, Washington, DC

One case in particular made me aware of the existence of secondary traumatic stress. I saw a seven-year-old girl who lived with her adoptive mother. She ran to a neighbor's home one day and told the neighbor that her mother was going to kill her. This neighbor called for help. Eventually, the young girl came to see me. She was emaciated and had scars upon scars upon scars. She talked about being locked in a room and tortured. She also told me she had a brother who she said was in the hospital.

After seeing her, I went back to my office to write up my report. I called the detective to tell him of my findings. He was still at the crime scene. He sounded shaken. He told me they had found her brother in the home. He was dead.

That evening, I was in bed talking to my husband and I said to him, "You know, maybe we could adopt her." He politely said, "No." We both knew it was not a good idea to bring work home like that. For a while after seeing her, I would dream about her. Our staff gave her some jewelry. Later she left a piece with me. I still have it hanging in my office.

I became quite attached to her while she was in the hospital. She became attached to me as well. When she would return for therapy, she would ask to see me. For whatever reason, I was usually not around. After a while, I realized that was for the best. I needed to keep some separation. The best I could do to help her was to do my job, write an objective and comprehensive report, and testify in court.

I once wrote an essay with a colleague of mine about secondary trauma and the lack of support systems for professionals who do this kind of work. Even though it was never published, writing it was therapeutic.

We all get the question. "How do you do this work?" I purge on paper. I remember these extreme cases, but most cases are out of my mind very quickly once I write the report. I find myself fully engaged when evaluating a child and writing a report. But once I am done, I leave that case and move onto the next one.

### Martin Finkel, DO, Stratford, New Jersey

There are some days when I walk out of the office shaking my head thinking, "How did I get through such a difficult day?" Yet, that feeling is invariably counterbalanced by a sense of great accomplishment.

I believe that one of the keys to survival in this field is being able to reflect, as opposed to absorb, all the emotional energy from the stories we hear of traumatized children. I tell my residents, "If you had a bleeding laceration and the emergency room doctor fainted when they saw it, would you have any confidence in that doctor?" Of course you wouldn't.

So we have to figure out how to process this stuff in a way that is healthy, not just for ourselves, but for the children we see. If you can't figure out how to do that, you won't be in this field very long.

When I give lectures, I always use cases to make a point. Sometimes the case material is hard to listen to, sometimes it is uplifting. I spoke to a child once who was having difficulty talking about what had happened to her. Finally, she opened up and said, "I can tell you because you're my doctor." It was such a simple statement, but it was so amazing and uplifting to have that child, for whatever reason, feel comfortable sharing her story with me.

### Stephen C. Boos, MD, Springfield, Massachusetts

I saw an infant with an unusual bruise on his hand that the family seemed able to explain. I did a full abuse workup and found no additional injuries.

Three months later, his mother brought him back to the emergency room for some reason, but then they left before he could be seen. He apparently was fine in the waiting room. His mom had taken a video of him playing.

He came back dead several hours later. He had extensive brain injury and many old and new rib fractures. Did I miss something? Did I do enough?

In another case, I was called to the ER to see a little girl who had old and new whipping injuries on her back. She also had an untreated elbow fracture that left her with a permanent deformity. She had been beaten by her father. It was easy enough to advocate for that child's safety. Eventually she was placed with her grandmother.

She would come in to see one of our therapists on a regular basis and she bonded with me. I got to see her a lot, to see the positive changes in her life. It was very gratifying.

So here are two stories, one positive one and one negative. Both are always going to stay with me.

People always ask me, "How can you do this work?" What they're really asking is how can you see what's happening to these children and live with the emotions. That's never been an issue for me. The issue for me has always been the receiver operator curve (a curve that assesses the likelihood of a correct diagnosis), the balance between alpha and beta error (the balance between making the correct diagnosis and making the wrong one). Perhaps more than most of my colleagues, I see the world as a probability distribution within which we have to make decisions. We have to take action. Sometimes we get it wrong.

### Marcellina Mian, MDCM, MPHE, Qatar

There is a case that haunts me to this day. A three-year-old boy suffered from failure to thrive. His parents had cognitive limitations and were unemployed. They also were drinkers. But they were doing the best they could under the circumstances. They were getting a lot of community support.

But then, a second child was born who also suffered from failure to thrive. For CPS, this was the last straw and both children were taken into custody.

I distinctly remember the scene at the courthouse. The three-year-old literally had to be peeled off of his mother's body. It was terrible. I really felt that, despite their risk factors, these parents loved their children and would never have harmed them.

I saw the three-year-old in follow-up. He was in foster care. His weight had gone up. He was doing better. The foster father said to me, "You know, one of the problems we have is that CPS stipulates that we cannot use corporal punishment. We cannot spank this child. We spank our other children." I told him, "Treat him the way you would treat your own children." A few months later, this child was killed when his foster parent threw him down a flight of stairs. I testified at the murder trial.

As I said, this case haunts me. His parents would never have harmed him. I also wonder what would have happened had I given the foster father advice around discipline that did not involve corporal punishment.

### Alice W. Newton, MD, Boston, Massachusetts

Working in child abuse can be challenging, not only because of the many sad stories but because of the public controversies about abuse. The debate about abusive head trauma came to Boston in 2016 and I decided to respond publically. I knew that there could be repercussions from working with the press, but I felt that telling my story was the right thing to do, because the defense argument about this issue is so inaccurate.

In Boston, we had three cases in a row that the medical examiner originally diagnosed as abuse then re-diagnosed as not abuse. My opinion was that the medical examiner had been influenced by a handful of defense witnesses, as well as by some of the controversial forensic pathology literature that questions the existence of abusive head trauma. I made the decision to take that issue on by working closely with an excellent reporter from the *Boston Globe*.

At the same time, there was a very public case of medical child abuse involving a girl whom I cared for at another hospital. The blowback from conservative press and child abuse naysayers was intense. I was personally attacked. I received death threats on Facebook. The state police had to visit my home, talk to my children, and make sure my home was secure. It was very stressful for me and my family.

I still would make the same decision. Patty Wen, the reporter from the *Boston Globe*, and I worked closely together. We did a story about what child abuse pediatrics is all about. She wrote other excellent pieces which covered the medical examiner controversy.

How can I still do this work despite these stresses? I remember a four-year-old little boy who came in to see me. His mother was a drug addict and she had left him and his sister with their addict aunt, while she partied over the weekend. When their mother came back to get them, her son had a broken leg and tons of bruises. He told us that he had been beaten with a broom stick and needles had been stuck under his fingernails.

The case was so horrible. It was one of the few times I actually used the word "torture." In the hospital, his foster family came in with their children and a photo album of everyone. It was just the sweetest thing. Eventually his mother lost custody of him and he was adopted by this family. That's the kind of nice story that gives me hope.

Despite the difficulties of the work, the terrible abuse, the professional conflicts, the workplace stresses, having my worldview altered was never a problem for me. My own cognitive schema, forged during my inner-city childhood, was that the world was always unsafe, always terrifying. Even so, even after all these years, there are cases that still horrify me.

## About Megan

Megan was 14 months old when I saw her in the hospital. She had extensive bruising of her face, neck, mouth, throat, chest, and back. Despite the absence of life-threating injuries, the story of how she was injured and how she got to the hospital was one of the most harrowing I have ever heard. It was also the first and only time I have ever felt physically ill interviewing a parent.

On the morning Megan was eventually hospitalized, she awoke in her crib while her mother Cheryl and her mother's boyfriend Bruce slept in. They had been drinking the night before. Megan was used to being alone and awake in the morning in her crib. She never cried out, even if she were wet or hungry.

Cheryl's sleep was interrupted by a phone call from a relative who needed a ride to the doctor's office. Her car had broken down and she begged Cheryl for help. Reluctantly, Cheryl got up, woke a very unhappy Bruce, dressed Megan, and placed her in her car seat. Before leaving to pick up the friend, Cheryl and Bruce each downed two shots of coffee brandy. Then they got in the car with Megan, left the two older school age children at home, and drove to pick up the friend.

In the doctor's parking lot, Cheryl, Bruce, and Megan waited for the friend to come out. Megan had not eaten nor had she been changed, and now some hours into the morning she began to whine in the back seat of the car. Bruce was seen by a passerby reaching back and backhanding Megan several times across her face. He also was seen grabbing her by the collar and boxing her ears. Obviously, each blow only made Megan cry more so that the next blow was even harder than the one before. The passerby also saw Cheryl and Bruce drinking in the car.

The horrified passerby told a security guard at the doctor's office what he had seen. The security guard called the police. Before the police arrived, the passerby left, although he came forward later when the full extent of Megan's injuries was reported in the news. It was never clear what the police were told. Were they told that Megan had been hit several times in the face? Were they told that Cheryl and Bruce were seen drinking in the car?

Whatever they were told, they never looked at Megan. If they had, they would have certainly seen her facial injuries, if not the new ones that were just starting to develop, then the older ones there from being hit days earlier by either Bruce or Cheryl or both.

Apparently, the police were only interested in the drinking. They gave Bruce and Cheryl a field sobriety test, which they failed. Then they left after telling them to have the friend drive the car when she came out of the office. The police did not notify child protective services that a child was in the car with two drunken adults.

Eventually the family made its way back home. No one knows who drove. Later in the afternoon, another relative came to the house to see Megan. She became concerned when neither Cheryl nor Bruce would answer the door. The door was unlocked so she entered to find Cheryl and Bruce passed out on their bed with Megan sitting on her mother's chest screaming. She saw Megan's bruised and bloodied face. She asked Cheryl where the bruises had come from. Cheryl replied, "What bruises? There aren't any bruises." The relative scooped Megan up and rushed her to the hospital.

Luckily, other than the extensive bruising, Megan was medically, though certainly not psychologically, OK. There was old and new bruising of both ears. There was bruising of both sides of her face, worse on the right, consistent with the report of the witness of a right-hand backhanding the child's face. She also had older grab mark bruises on her back and ligature like marks on the back of her neck as if she had been grabbed by her shirt. Her lips were swollen and bruised and there was extensive bruising of the back of her throat. All the injuries both old and new could be explained by blows to the face and grabbing of the trunk, all except the bruising of the back of the throat which was never explained. Could this have represented a pacifier or cup or spoon jammed into her mouth? Could it have been something worse? Even after a plea bargain was reached with Bruce and he was sentenced, no one bothered to ask him how the bruising of the throat had happened.

Megan had no internal injuries, no head trauma, and no abdominal trauma. It was a near thing though. How many of her injuries occurred after the police saw the family will never be known. Certainly, given the severity of the injuries she did have, further injury could have been fatal.

Megan was taken into CPS custody and placed in foster care. It was some days after this that I had an opportunity to interview her mother. Cheryl answered all of my questions without hesitation, without emotion, and without any remorse. She never once asked me how Megan was doing. Seeing Megan's injuries, photographing them, knowing she had been abused multiple times, was very much a clinical rather than an emotional issue for me. The emotional difficulty for me came when I listened to Cheryl's matter-of-fact, almost cold-blooded, retelling of what had happened that day.

What was most odd was how Cheryl looked or didn't look. She did not look impaired. She was neatly dressed and answered my questions directly and easily. She did not hesitate or appear to cover up anything. That might be a sign of cooperation. But neither did she show any emotion, not a tear, or a catch in her voice. It was almost as if she were telling me a story about some other family.

Cheryl told me that she "woke to a phone call from a friend who needed a ride." Bruce was still asleep. She woke him, then both of them "downed two shots of coffee brandy each." They got Megan dressed and put her in the car, then they drove to pick up the friend. On the way they "continued to drink coffee brandy." While waiting for the friend outside the doctor's office, they "drank some more." At this point, I counted five to six shots of coffee brandy each. It was still morning and they were driving with the baby in the back of the car.

I stopped her at this point. I wanted to know more of what happened that day but first I needed to know more about Cheryl and Bruce. She told me they were both in their twenties. Neither of them worked. Bruce, according to Cheryl, was "an alcoholic." Cheryl told me that she had a history of cocaine and opiate abuse "but not in the last six months." They had been together for about five months and despite the injuries to Megan were still together. She had no plans to separate from him since "he hadn't done anything wrong."

She did tell me that Bruce could be violent "but only when he drank." She failed to add that he, and indeed she, drank all the time. The relative who I spoke to later told me that they drank between them a half a gallon of liquor a day. Cheryl also knew that he was on the sex offender registry and was not allowed to see his own children, but that was all "just a misunderstanding."

Cheryl then continued with her story of that day. In the parking lot, still drinking, with Megan whining in the back seat, a knock on the window interrupted them. It was the police who asked them to step out of the car for a field sobriety test. According to Cheryl, they both failed and agreed to let their friend drive them home.

Cheryl seemed unable or unwilling to tell me what happened after that. She told me that much of the day was a blur because of the drinking. She did know that someone had said they had seen Bruce hit Megan in the parking lot but she said it didn't happen. She did tell me that Megan had bruising on both ears a few days earlier and that she had planned on taking her to see her doctor "in a few days."

The relative who saved Megan told me that she had long had concerns about Cheryl and Bruce and their drinking. She had actually cared for Megan for six months because of Cheryl's ongoing problem with alcohol and drugs. She had even called child protective services but had gotten no response.

As I was talking to Cheryl, I could feel myself getting more and more upset. Maybe it was anger, maybe it was sadness, but whatever it was, I could not get the image out of my head of Megan crying forlornly as she lay on top of her passed out mother.

This normally does not happen to me. I don't normally visualize the scene where the abuse happened. But here was something so visceral, so immediate, and so palpable that I could not get let go of that image for many days. Every time I thought of Megan on her mother's chest, I felt a rush of adrenalin sometimes associated with nausea but always associated with the intrusive image of that scene.

It wasn't the physical abuse, or the drinking, or even Cheryl's blank apathetic stare that made me recoil. It was this vivid image encapsulating in one sudden scene all that was wrong with this mother, all the damage she had done to her child by not protecting her from abuse, maybe by even abusing her herself. It was the beautiful book of photography *The Family of Man* turned inside out.

I almost wished I had an actual picture. Perhaps then I would not be imagining Cheryl splayed out on the bed, drooling out of the side of her mouth, dirty sheets and pillows tossed asunder, the stench of alcohol and vomit and dirty diapers and spoiled food, Bruce next to her snoring loudly in his disheveled clothing, the floor impassable because of littered clothing, empty and partially empty bottles of alcohol scattered on the floor, bureau drawers half open with clothing hanging out, dirt everywhere, peeling paint, dirty windows, torn shades, and above it all the terrible wail of a baby with nowhere to turn to for help except the warm body of her passed out mother.

The entire time I was interviewing Cheryl, I was seeing Megan in that home. This is not what a scene from a home should look like. I wanted so much to tell her what I thought of her actions. I wanted so much to scream at her, to somehow shake her out of her apathy and ignorance, to make her understand what horrible things she had done. I could not do that however. As always, my job was to gather information, not stifle it by criticism. And so I sat there, my hand over my mouth as a precaution against speaking, all the while feeling sicker and sicker.

The contrast between that horrific image and the banal mother sitting in front of me was more than I could ever understand. It took me many days of telling and retelling that story to colleagues to gain some perspective, to finally disengage from that scene.

As much as I felt anger mingled with so many other emotions about what had been done to Megan, I don't think I ever felt directly angry with Cheryl. She was, in so many ways, a victim of her own life, limited in personal resources, unable to surmount any of the many obstacles in her way.

I am often asked by students why some parents seem to hook up over and over again with alcoholics, with drug abusers, with batterers, with sex offenders. I know the answer is multifaceted and complex. But sometimes I think that, in the dysfunctional, often economically and resource poor communities where these parents live, there are no other choices. Their choices are limited to alcoholics, sex offenders, batterers, and child abusers. I can feel pity in those circumstances and certainly in some ways felt pity for Cheryl.

Maybe that is how I finally came to terms with Megan's story, by seeing Cheryl as the end product of her unfortunate circumstances, starting perhaps even before she was born, probably in her childhood, and certainly in her current living environment. We all make choices in our lives. For some of us, the range of choices is broad, for others, like Cheryl, the choices are all limited and all bad. At least now, Megan, protected in a safe environment, is no longer a part of those choices.

So, how do we continue to do the work?

In his book *Homicide: A Year on the Killing Street*, David Simon (1991) wrote: "For each body, he gives what he can afford to give and no more. He carefully measures out the required amount of energy and emotion, closes the file and moves on to the next call. And even after years of calls and bodies and crime scenes and interrogations, a good detective still answers the phone with the stubborn, unyielding belief that if he does his job, the truth is always knowable. A homicide detective endures."

This is a work ethic many child abuse pediatricians would agree with.

This chapter marks the end of child abuse stories, apart from the epilogue that finally answers the question of what really happened in the woodshed. The next chapter is made up of the voices of child abuse pediatricians talking about the future of child abuse pediatrics and about what it will take to keep our children safe from abuse.

## CHAPTER TEN

# The Future of Our Children: Child Abuse Prevention in America and Internationally

So far this book has been about case stories as a window into the secret lives of battered children. This final chapter is simply the voices of child abuse pediatricians talking about the future of our field, the future of child abuse prevention in our country, and the future of international prevention, essentially the future of our children.

## International Efforts to Treat and Prevent Child Abuse

### Sabine Ann Maguire, MBBCh, BAO, Cardiff, Wales, United Kingdom

It's important to point out that clinical child abuse in the United Kingdom is not a subspecialty like it is in the United States. It was decided that if you specialize in child abuse here, you did so while practicing community pediatrics. I think this system has merits. You can keep perspective because you see a lot of normal children with normal childhood illnesses. On the other hand, there should be a minimum level of child abuse work that you do to be sufficiently expert.

Having worked with some American child abuse pediatricians, I can see the attraction of the American system of specialization. They do gain a lot of expertise, but perhaps risk losing wider general pediatric knowledge and experience. I think that as long as you have a minimum amount of child abuse pediatric experience (two to three days a week at least), the U.K. model is probably a good one.

On the other hand, our emergency room physicians, who see little abuse, are patchy in their ability to correctly identify it. This is not just a problem here; it is also an issue in U.S. hospitals. Studies have shown that there is quite a drop off in skill level outside of pediatric hospitals.

In 2002, we began conducting systematic reviews to look at the investigation of suspected abusive injuries. Originally, the work was intended to look only at bruising. But then it became clear that systematic reviews would be helpful to medical providers who were evaluating all sorts of injuries for abuse.

Much of my work has been in developing guidance for the United Kingdom based on our systematic reviews. We developed the first comprehensive training program for all pediatricians in the United Kingdom.

Overall, I think there's more consistent practice now. In the past, individual practitioners developed their own approach and stuck rigidly to what they called abuse and what they didn't call abuse. I still find reluctance among pediatricians internationally to change their practice if the evidence doesn't agree with them. One example of this is the reluctance to accept the research findings that aging bruises from visual inspection is quite imprecise. Another area where new literature contradicts older practice is with regard to spiral fractures of the femur in toddlers. We now know from published research that such fractures are often accidental.

Since the mid-2000s, there's been a substantial improvement in the quality of research. Overall I would say that the availability of high-quality research has led to a more consistent approach to the diagnosis of abuse.

One thing that is problematic in the United Kingdom is the view that the press has about abuse. Their opinion is either that pediatricians and social workers are over-calling abuse and unnecessarily taking children from their parents or that these professionals are allowing children to stay in abusive homes where they then die.

Professionals in the United Kingdom are vilified, photographed, and followed. I have been targeted personally. I have had to change my car license plate number. I have had to have physical protection. It is almost like a witch hunt. The U.K. press never seems to report on a good story where a child was correctly identified and either saved from removal or saved from death.

Families have been encouraged by various groups to file formal complaints with the General Medical Council if we diagnose abuse. The fact that we don't have mandatory reporting laws in the United Kingdom makes it more difficult for us by removing the layer of protection for reporting that the Unites States has. All of this makes it very stressful to work in the United Kingdom.

I believe we have improved the plight of children, particularly in the last 10 years, by increasing our focus on neglect and emotional abuse. In particular, educational staff are more comfortable reporting cases of neglect and emotional abuse. The fact that all of our younger doctors undergo mandatory child protection training means that they are more confident in their ability to recognize and refer children who have been abused.

Unfortunately, at the same time, because of cost cuts, there has been a reduction in the level of training that social workers get on the medical aspects of child abuse. We have done research that shows that our social workers have limited knowledge about physical abuse-related injuries. Since the average length of time social workers stay in the field is 21 months, by the time they gain that knowledge from experience, they have moved on.

I also think we need to increase our focus on parental readiness by targeting school children and fathers. One in ten fathers have postnatal depression and we still don't screen for it.

### Jocelyn Brown, MD, MPH, New York

Currently, I have two international projects, one in France, and one in Cuba.

The French project is a partnership between the Mailman School of Public Health at Columbia University and the School of Public Health in France (Ecole des Hautes Etudes en Sante Publique or EHESP). This project is a comparative study of the role of school physicians in child abuse identification and reporting. France does not have child abuse pediatric specialists. I go to France once a year to train future school physicians about sexual abuse.

I think doctors in France don't want to report child abuse or they want to report in such a way that they know the family is going to benefit from the report. One of the interesting things about the French child welfare system is that it resembles our differential response, also known in New York as Family Assessment Response (FAR). (Differential response means that higher severity cases receive a child protective assessment, while lower severity cases receive in-home support services.) Child Advocacy Centers are slowly emerging. They are based within university teaching hospitals and called "Unites medico-legales."

Cuba is interesting. I go to Cuba to teach about abuse. They have a strong medical system rooted in the community, in the neighborhood. I believe that any system hoping to protect children and families has to be rooted in the community. The Cuban health-care system is integrated into the community. Every neighborhood has a family doctor and nurse team who live in the community. They treat the entire family. They know the strengths and weaknesses of the families they see. Data are regularly collected at the neighborhood level to inform the medical providers. As a result, health-risk factors are known and can be treated. There are also mental health professionals available for the families. Doctors make house calls. Pregnant mothers get more prenatal visits than in the Unites States and Cuba's infant mortality rate is lower than in the Unites States.

We should try to learn from successes in these two countries.

## Gabriel Otterman, MD, Uppsala, Sweden

I practice in the field of child abuse pediatrics at Uppsala University Children's Hospital, an academic teaching hospital north of Stockholm. We have a team that performs inpatient and outpatient clinical consults. We also have a foster care clinic. It's the first foster care clinic in Sweden. It's a medical home for children in out-of-home care that provides both intake evaluations and follow-up visits.

I cochair the section on Child Maltreatment in the Swedish Pediatric Society. We have a network of 130 pediatricians around the country who engage in some way in this area of practice. I feel strengthened and supported by this network of professionals.

Sweden is a wonderful country. It has done great things for child rights. In 1979, Sweden was the first country to ban corporal punishment. Many factors make the social determinants of health a lot better in Sweden than in the Unites States. The social welfare system is robust. There is generous parental leave along with high-quality daycare and early childhood education.

One of the challenges for us in Europe is communication and collaboration across countries. The Unites States has child fatality review committees in all of the states with collaboration between states. Very few countries in Europe have that.

## Desmond K. Runyan, MD, DrPH, Denver, Colorado

In 1984, I was teaching a clinical epidemiology course for medical students at the University of North Carolina. The chairperson from the

Department of Preventative Medicine from the University of Alexandria, Egypt, came to one of my lectures. Afterward, she invited me to come to Alexandria to teach. I was there for three weeks teaching medical residents about clinical epidemiology.

One day, we were talking about my child abuse research and a student said, "Child abuse doesn't happen here in Egypt." I knew that couldn't be true but I didn't have the research to back it up.

Three years later, I was lecturing in Chile about abuse and one of the professors said that child abuse didn't happen in Chile. By then, there was some international research. I told him that there was data to suggest otherwise. He insisted that child abuse only happened in the United States. When I asked him how he knew that, he said, "Because all of the articles about abuse come from the U.S."

A year later, I met with people from 15 different countries to develop a common questionnaire for families to study harsh discipline patterns. That project developed new and useful cross-cultural data on child discipline. The results showed, among other things, that Chile and Egypt had a more serious problem than the Unites States.

Subsequently, I initiated, with a much larger group of investigators, the development of new measurement tools for discipline and abuse designed to be explicitly cross-cultural. These tools were called the ICAST instruments (International Society for the Prevention of Child Abuse and Neglect Child Abuse Screening Tool). They included a parent questionnaire, a child questionnaire, and a youth retrospective questionnaire, that ask about physical and emotional discipline, neglect, and sexual abuse. These instruments are now or have already been used in 83 countries.

One of the findings of this international research is that less maternal education is one of the strongest predictors of harsh discipline. Internationally, girls' education makes a huge difference, not only in rates of harsh discipline but in rates of children under the age of two being shaken.

One of my conclusions from this work is that educating girls around the world would reduce the burden of child maltreatment more than almost anything else we could do. Educated mothers talk to their children more and consequently their children have better language development. Educated mothers also delay child bearing, so they are more mature when they do have children.

### Marcellina Mian, MDCM, MPHE, Qatar

I am writing up the results of a study on the nature and extent of child discipline in two Arab countries using the ICAST parent and youth retrospective questionnaires. It was a difficult study to do because no one wants to talk about child abuse in emerging countries. That is not the image these countries want to show the world.

In international research, there is also the problem of differing definitions of what constitutes child abuse. I once saw a nine-year-old girl who was badly beaten by her father. Identifying what was done and who had done it was not the problem. The father said he did it. He also said, "She went to the neighbor's house. She wasn't supposed to do that. It made it look as though I don't look after my children. She needed to be beaten." This happened in a society where family honor is of great importance. The daughter's behavior reflected on her family's honor.

Sexual abuse is something that nobody wants to talk about, especially in countries where sex itself is a taboo subject. A case which really spoke to me about the issues was that of a nine-year-old boy who had been sexually abused by a neighbor. The abuse came to light because he had sustained some injuries. The father didn't want to involve the authorities. He said, "If I have to bring this out in the open, if I have to report this, then I have to kill my son and I have to kill the neighbor. I don't want to do that." Here again, family honor was of paramount importance. To protect his son, the father prevented him from ever again being alone with the neighbor.

### Aaron J. Miller, MD, MPA, New York

My interest is in developing the capacity of health systems across the world to address child maltreatment as a public health issue.

In 2008, I was director of the Lincoln Child Advocacy Center in New York. I was also studying for a MPA on International Development at Columbia University. One of my classmates ran a small foundation helping farmers in Malawi buy fertilizer to increase corn crop yield. We were out having drinks at the end of a long day and I told him I was director of a child abuse treatment center in the Bronx. He said, "If you design a program for Malawi, I will fund it."

Five months later, I was in Malawi with a child abuse prosecutor and a social worker. For two days, we trained 45 Malawian doctors, nurses, social workers, police, and a magistrate on the diagnosis and treatment of sexual abuse, physical abuse, and intimate partner violence.

During this same trip, UNICEF (United Nations Children's Fund) arranged a stakeholder meeting to discuss the creation of 20 one-stop centers for treatment of child maltreatment and intimate partner violence. Police and Social Welfare had been working with UNICEF to plan the centers, but there had not been any outreach to the health sector. The stakeholder meeting included 14 leaders from the Ministries of Social Welfare, Police and Health. By the end of the meeting, the group decided that all these centers should be based at hospitals. Now eight years later, Malawi has 20 hospital-based one-stop centers, 9 of them have received training from members of the Ray Helfer Society.

I recently worked in Namibia. The country has 14 violence protection units that are akin to law enforcement-based child advocacy centers in the United States. UNICEF hired me to help develop standard operating procedures for the centers and to provide a training of trainers to the leaders of these centers to improve the diagnosis and treatment of sexual and physical violence. At two of the centers, I will provide extra mentoring. I will be in the room when they take the medical history and perform a medical exam. I will also assist them in improving case review and follow-up.

## The Future of Child Welfare and Child Abuse Pediatrics in America

### Richard Krugman, MD, Aurora, Colorado

Henry Kempe had a big impact on my work in this field. He was doing stuff in the early 1970s around prevention that no one else was doing. He put a video camera in the delivery room at Colorado General and, with parent permission, videotaped 150 consecutive deliveries. He was examining the parent-child interaction at the time of delivery.

He found that 80 percent of the 150 families were happy and excited about their baby. But 20 percent clearly were not. They wouldn't hold the baby and would make comments like, "the baby is ugly. He looks like the guy who raped me." There were other behaviors and statements that suggested these families might be at risk.

But Henry didn't just watch. He developed one of the earliest home visitation programs in the country. Half the high-risk families were assigned to have home visitation. The other half were not. Two years later, the results showed that the home visitation families had not a single episode of abuse while, of the families that did not get services, five had cases of abuse. That study showed that if you give help to families, particularly those at high risk, you can make a difference.

### Stephen C. Boos, MD, FAAP, Springfield, Massachusetts

I think that our individual clinical practice needs to include prevention, support for foster children, and assuring that children and families get appropriate treatment. Prevention isn't just about telling people not to shake babies and then hoping they don't shake their babies. Prevention should be rooted in child development and behavior.

I once read a book called *Parent Making*. It was about making us good parents. I think that's where prevention lies. I think it lies in parent making and advocating for families at risk and dealing with children's behavioral challenges before it's too late. I think that this is an area where child abuse pediatrics needs to reintegrate with child behavioral health, so we can take care of these families before they abuse their children.

## Desmond K. Runyan, MD, DrPH, Denver, Colorado

My focus is on trying to increase the amount of research and research funding in the field. Three million children a year are reported to child protective services. Of these, several hundred thousand are substantiated as having been abused. Yet, the overall funding for child abuse research is only $30 million a year in this country.

My data suggests that 6 percent of Colorado children were physically abused last year. If the data from other states suggests that 1 percent were sexually abused and another 4 or 5 percent were neglected, that means that 8 or 9 percent, almost 1 in 10 of our children, are abused each year in this country. Official child welfare statistics don't come anywhere near capturing all of these children.

## John M. Leventhal, MD, New Haven, Connecticut

What I would like to see in Connecticut is for every emergency department to have a child abuse team connected to an academic center and connected to child protective services. I think this would link the healthcare and the CPS systems in a much more powerful, positive way. We are now piloting this linkage system in a few hospitals in the state.

I also think we need more child abuse doctors who focus their research and clinical activities on prevention. It is not enough to help children and families after the maltreatment has occurred. The field needs to work on developing and testing better prevention programs and more nurturing communities, so fewer children suffer from abuse and neglect.

## Suzanne P. Starling, MD, San Diego, California

Recently, when I was on call, I went into the hospital for what I call "a mercy call." I was seeing a baby with a linear skull fracture. The medical staff was convinced that the injury and history didn't match and were preparing to discharge the child into foster care.

The story was that the baby had fallen off the ottoman. The medical staff thought that was not an adequate explanation for a skull fracture. To me, it was a great explanation for this baby's injury. I was able to tell the police and the child protective worker that the described fall from an ottoman could certainly have caused the linear skull fracture. I told them that the child was not abused and did not need to go into foster care. When I explained the situation to the family, the baby's grandmother hugged me so hard I thought she would break one of my ribs.

My interest is in quality improvement in our field and particularly in trying to get providers steered toward similar diagnostic criteria. The ultimate goal would be to eliminate some of the diagnostic variability in the field.

## Cindy W. Christian, MD, Philadelphia, Pennsylvania

I was the medical director for a child welfare agency for five years. The work was both rewarding and frustrating. The child welfare administration was incredibly supportive and welcoming. They recognized the benefits of having a health-care provider working in their agency. But the workers and supervisors were not always as embracing.

When I first got there, I thought it would be wise to meet with a small group of case workers and administrators to talk about their complex medical cases. I thought that would be a great place to start a relationship. I e-mailed them to set up a meeting. I got an e-mail back telling me they were too busy to meet, not too busy to meet anytime soon, but too busy to meet at all, ever.

At the time, I had been working at the Children's Hospital of Philadelphia for more than 25 years. I had never had a situation where I asked someone to meet and they said, "No, I'm too busy." I have had people say, and I myself have said, that now is not a good time, but let's meet later. These workers and supervisors were basically saying to me, "No, we don't really want you here. We don't see your value to us."

I did have some successes working with that agency. For example, when I started there, they had two nurses making home visits. When I left, there were eleven. That was one of our greatest accomplishments.

I believe it is time for the medical community, all of us, to show that we can actually improve the health of children in foster care. It should be our goal to make sure that, when children leave the system, they are healthier than when they arrived.

We also need to support parents, particularly those with children who have behavioral problems. But it is going to take more than child abuse pediatricians. It is going to take a society that recognizes that families need help and a society willing to provide it to them. We are talking here about impoverished families, families with mental health issues, families where there is unemployment and limited education. At the core of all of these issues is crushing poverty, one of the most powerful predictors of child abuse in this country.

### Christopher S. Greeley, MD, MS, Houston, Texas

We started a section called Public Health Pediatrics at Baylor College of Medicine and Texas Children's Hospital. I have this vision of wanting to do more with adversity and resilience and social determinants of health. We developed community-based strategies for different child adversities such as postpartum depression, intimate partner violence, and food insecurity. We also do abusive head trauma prevention. Our framework is public health—community-based, collaborative, capacity building, the three Cs of our section. One of our goals is to decrease child abuse, but we also have a goal of improving child and family well-being.

The world is an unfair place, but it doesn't have to be. It has sharp edges, but those sharp edges can be filed down and made less sharp. My personal belief is that we have to go upstream and identify at-risk families before bad things happen to them.

I think that child abuse pediatricians are the only ones who are positioned to do this work. We care for those at the tip of the spear. We have the compelling arguments, we have the framework, and we have the motivation.

I was a young assistant professor at Vanderbilt. My wife was a pediatrician there as well. Quite unexpectedly, we had triplet boys. We were struggling academic pediatricians. I was moonlighting to save money. The date was February 19, 2005. I remember the day specifically. It was 10 o'clock at night and one of my boys had colic. He was three-months-old and he was crying and crying and crying. I was so stressed and so tired. I remember picking him up, looking at his face, and saying to myself, "Now I understand. Now I know how good people could do something horrible to their child." Nothing bad happened, but that was, in part, because I had a very bright and compassionate wife and a supportive family.

That experience really triggered something in me. I no longer feel angry or frustrated with parents who abuse their children. I just feel sad.

For the most part, these parents are not evil people who wake up wanting to hurt their children. These are parents who are struggling, parents who reach a breaking point. After that experience, I became more involved with prevention. I was on the board of Prevent Child Abuse Tennessee and then on the board of Prevent Child Abuse America. I started focusing on the question of what gets people to the point of injuring their child.

One of the most compelling conversations I ever had on this topic was with the dean of the Education School at Vanderbilt. He was interested in child abuse. I told him I was interested in preventing child abuse. He said to me, "Mom raises her hand. She's about to strike her child. Our response is to go in there and grab her and prevent her from hitting her child. What I'm interested in is why did mom think she had to raise her hand in the first place?" That comment really helped me understand the problem.

I see prevention as fairly broad. To me postpartum depression screening is a child abuse prevention strategy. Job training is a child abuse prevention strategy. Keeping young women in school is a child abuse prevention strategy.

As a prevention strategy, Nurse-Family Partnership is quite good. So is Healthy Families America, Parents as Teachers, Safe Care, and Triple P. Triple P is an example of a program where parent support is tiered. Everyone gets some support, but the greatest amount of support is given to the highest-risk families. That's a strategy.

# Epilogue: Strider: What Happened in the Woodshed!

This book started with a question. What happened to Danny in that woodshed? It ends with a story about Strider, a young boy who survived a vicious beating in a woodshed.

Strider's story tells us not only what happened to Strider but what likely happened to Danny. It also tells us about the experience of so many abused and neglected children in our country. In that telling, perhaps we can gain some insight into the secret lives of battered children and perhaps we can gain some insight into how to better protect and nurture our children.

Strider's story is recreated here from newspaper and public court reports.

At two-and-a-half, Strider was a normal, active toddler who sometimes didn't finish his dinner and sometimes wet his pants. Everything was going along fine, that is, until his mother Heather brought home Justin, her new boyfriend. Then everything changed.

Heather and three of her children, ages 11 months (Gallager), 2 years (Strider), and a 7-year-old, lived in a mobile home with Justin. Over the next two months, Strider often had bruises on his face and buttocks. Justin always had an explanation. "He fell off the couch." "He fell in the bushes."

Then the swearing and the threats started.

"Shut the fuck up Strider."

"He's a fucking crybaby."

"You should just drown him."

One evening they all sat down to dinner. Justin became angry with Strider, because he didn't want to eat, and sent him to bed.

After dinner, Justin went outside to his woodshed to work and drink. Heather and the children went to bed. Heather awoke around 2 A.M. to find that Strider was not in his bed. She got up and found him in the shed with Justin. It was a bitterly cold night. Strider was wrapped in a blanket and sleeping in a chair. Justin mumbled something about teaching him or breaking him. She asked Justin to bring Strider back into the house then she went back to bed.

Around 4 A.M., she awoke again. Strider was still not in his bed. She went out and tried to enter the shed, but this time Justin would not let her in. He had covered the windows so she could not see in. Heather again went back inside.

Finally, around 5 A.M., Justin brought Strider, now naked except for a diaper, back into the trailer. Justin then woke all the children. He screamed at them, particularly the 11-month-old Gallager. He told them that waking them was payback for all the times they had woken him early in the morning. Justin jumped on the seven-year-old laying on the couch, bruising his legs. He grabbed Strider and threw him to the floor.

Finally, having had enough, Heather took the children to her car and drove away. A couple of hours later, she arrived at her mother's house. She made several stops along the way. All the while, Strider lay bruised and silent in the backseat of her car. She even drove past the hospital that Strider eventually ended up at.

Enroute to her mother's, she told the seven-year-old not to tell anyone what had happened with Justin. For that, Heather was convicted of witness tampering and spent several months in jail.

At her mother's, Heather finally could see that Strider was not well. He was not responding. His eyes were rolling back in his head. He had bruises all over his body. She took particular note of swelling around his anus.

At 7:20 A.M., Heather called the hospital and told them she was bringing her son in because she believed he had been beaten. First though, she asked the hospital staff if the police had to be involved. She told them she was concerned about getting their belongings from the trailer.

She and Strider arrived at the hospital at 8 A.M. In the hospital waiting room, while Heather was talking to a receptionist, another nurse noticed Strider slumped over in a chair.

Strider was rushed into a trauma room. He was unresponsive, hypothermic (low body temperature), and hypotensive (low blood pressure). The medical staff thought he was dying, as indeed he was. After aggressive resuscitation though, Strider was stable enough to be transported by helicopter to a children's hospital.

At that second hospital, Strider was found to have injury to his brain, bruising of his neck, ears, abdomen, and swelling of his anus. His spleen had ruptured as had his intestines. His pancreas was crushed. Bowel material and blood had spilled into his abdomen. The surgeon estimated that Strider had lost 50 percent of his blood volume into his abdomen. The loss of 20 percent causes severe shock, 50 percent is almost always fatal.

Because of the heroic work of the surgical team, Stridor miraculously survived. He underwent multiple surgeries and stayed in the hospital for three weeks. After leaving the hospital, he had to be fed through a tube for a year.

The surgeon and child abuse doctor who testified at Justin's trial said that Strider's injuries were caused by multiple, vicious blows to his body, particularly to his abdomen. The surgeon stated, "I recently operated on a girl a year older than Strider who only wore a lap belt and was in a head-on collision when her father fell asleep. Both cars were going 60 miles an hour. Both she and Strider had similar abdominal injuries, but Strider's were far worse."

It was thought by the doctors that the anal injury was caused by the profound abdominal trauma Strider had experienced. This is a finding that has been described, for example, when a car rolls over a child's abdomen.

One of the pieces of evidence presented by the prosecution at trial was a text message from Justin to Heather. It read, "I'm done helping you raise your retarded fucking assholes. The smart thing to do would have been to drown them at birth. They are fucked up for life."

At the end of the trial, the jury deliberated for a scant two hours before returning a guilty verdict on all counts. Justin was sentenced to up to 55 years in prison.

Strider's seven-year-old half-brother was placed with his father. The two youngest, Strider and his infant brother Gallager were placed with their paternal grandparents. Medical providers, mental health providers, and child protective service workers continued to be involved, at least for a while. Eventually though, all the services ended.

Four years later, a major newspaper picked up Strider's story. He and his brother Gallager were still with their grandparents. The family was not doing well. They had been evicted from their trailer and were homeless, living hand to mouth, with multiple unpaid bills and no money. All the supports, initially put into place when the children were taken into custody, were nowhere to be found. Child protective services had long since moved on to other cases. Strider's and Gallager's grandparents, Lynette and Larry, suffered from significant medical problems. The boys' father visited but he had mental health problems, which Lynette blamed on abuse from her first husband. The family was barely surviving.

Even with all that, the boys were deeply loved and fiercely protected by Lynette and Larry. They did their best to take care of the children, because as Lynette put it, "family is family."

But for Strider and Gallager, the world was turning bleaker by the day. The crushing poverty the family lived under dragged them all down, that is until the newspaper article.

That one newspaper article changed everything. The community response was immediate and profound. A fund was set up for the children's needs. The family was given a home and their rent was paid. Most importantly, the children were getting services they had always so desperately needed.

I recently saw Strider's and Gallager's father and paternal grandparents in the hallway of a court house. Lynette and Larry were concluding their adoption of the boys. The future was bright. I was very happy for them.

As I was leaving the courthouse, Lynette showed me a mother's day poem Strider had written for her. I don't think I have ever read anything so moving. Good outcomes are possible for abused and neglected children in our country. It just takes a village with eyes and hearts wide open.

> My mom's name is Lynette.
> She is 61 years old.
> She has the same color eyes and hair that I do.
> She weighs 60, or 70, or 80 pounds and is 60, or 70, or 80 feet tall.
> She likes to try to get a chance to come outside.
> Her favorite food is tomato soup.
> My mom cooks the best tomato soup and grilled cheese!
> My mom really loves me and Gallager.
> My mom and I like to cook cake together. I got to help her make the cake.
> I love my mom because she loves me and Gallager
> Happy Mother's Day Mom!
> Love
> Strider

# Appendix:
# Child Abuse Doctors Who
# Shared Their Stories

Christine Barron, MD, FAAP
Associate Professor of Pediatrics and Clinical Educator
Warren Alpert Medical School of Brown University
Aubin Child Protection Center
Hasbro Children's Hospital
Providence, Rhode Island

Rachel P. Berger MD, MPH, FAAP
Professor of Pediatrics and Clinical and Translational Medicine
Children's Hospital of Pittsburgh of UPMC
Safar Center for Resuscitation Research
University of Pittsburgh
Pittsburgh, Pennsylvania

Robert W. Block, MD, FAAP
Past President, the American Academy of Pediatrics (2011–2012)
Chair and Professor Emeritus of Pediatrics, University of Oklahoma
Tulsa University School of Community Medicine
Tulsa, Oklahoma

Stephen C. Boos, MD, FAAP
Medical Director, Baystate Family Advocacy Center

Associate Professor of Pediatrics, Tufts University School of Medicine
Associate Professor of Pediatrics, University of Massachusetts Medical School
Springfield, Massachusetts

Jocelyn Brown, MD, MPH, FAAP
Professor of Pediatrics
Division of Child and Adolescent Health
Columbia University Medical Center
New York

Amanda Brownell, MD, FAAP
Child Abuse Fellow
Cincinnati Children's Hospital Medical Center
Cincinnati, Ohio

Cindy W. Christian, MD, FAAP
Anthony A. Latini Endowed Chair in Child Abuse and Neglect Prevention
Professor of Pediatrics
Associate Dean for Admissions
The Perelman School of Medicine at the University of Pennsylvania
The Children's Hospital of Philadelphia
Philadelphia, Pennsylvania

Howard Dubowitz, MD, MS, FAAP
Professor of Pediatrics
Head, Division of Child Protection
Director, Center for Families
Department of Pediatrics
University of Maryland School of Medicine
Baltimore, Maryland

Kenneth W. Feldman, MD, FAAP
Clinical Professor of Pediatrics
University of Washington School of Medicine
Children's Protection Program
Seattle Children's Hospital
Seattle, Washington

Martin A. Finkel, DO, FACOP, FAAP
Professor of Pediatrics
Medical Director, Institute Codirector
Child Abuse Research Education Service (CARES) Institute
Rowan University School of Osteopathic Medicine
Stratford, New Jersey

Emalee G. Flaherty, MD, FAAP
Professor Emeritus of Pediatrics
Northwestern Feinberg School of Medicine
Chicago, Illinois

Christopher S. Greeley, MD, MS, FAAP
Chief, Section of Public Health Pediatrics
Texas Children's Hospital
Vice-Chair for Community Health
Baylor College of Medicine
Houston, Texas

Kent P. Hymel, MD, FAAP
Professor of Pediatrics
Penn State College of Medicine
Department of Pediatrics
Division of Child Abuse Pediatrics
Milton S. Hershey Medical Center
Hershey, Pennsylvania

Allison M. Jackson, MD, MPH, FAAP
Division Chief, Freddie Mac Foundation Child & Adolescent Protection Center
Children's National Health Systems
Washington Children's Foundation Professor of Child & Adolescent Protection
Associate Professor of Pediatrics
The George Washington University School of Medicine and Health Sciences
Washington, DC

Carole Jenny, MD, MBA, FAAP
Professor of Pediatrics

University of Washington School of Medicine
Seattle Children's Hospital
Seattle, Washington

David Kerns, MD
Adjunct Clinical Professor of Pediatrics
Stanford University School of Medicine
Former Director, Center for Child Protection
Santa Clara Valley Medical Center
San Jose, California

Richard D. Krugman, MD, FAAP
Distinguished Professor of Pediatrics
University of Colorado School of Medicine
Kempe Center for the Prevention and Treatment of Child Abuse and Neglect
Aurora, Colorado

John M. Leventhal, MD, FAAP
Professor of Pediatrics
Yale School of Medicine
Director, Child Abuse Programs
Yale New Haven Children's Hospital
New Haven, Connecticut

Alex V. Levin, MD, MHSc, FRCSC FAAO, FAAP
Professor, Departments of Ophthalmology and Pediatrics
Sidney Kimmel Medical College at Thomas Jefferson University
Chief, Pediatric Ophthalmology and Ocular Genetics
Robison D. Harley, MD Endowed Chair in Pediatric Ophthalmology and Ocular
    Genetics
Wills Eye Hospital
Philadelphia, Pennsylvania

Sabine Ann Maguire, MBBCh, BAO, FRCPI, FRCPCH
Senior Research Fellow
School of Medicine
Cardiff University
Cardiff, Wales, United Kingdom

John McCann, MD, FAAP
Clinical Professor of Pediatrics, Retired
University of California School of Medicine
Davis, California

Marcellina Mian, MDCM, MPHE, FAAP
Professor Emerita of Pediatrics
Weill Cornell Medicine
Qatar

Aaron J. Miller, MD, MPA, FAAP
Executive Director, BRANCH (Building Regional Alliances to Nurture Child Health)
Assistant Professor of Clinical Pediatrics
Weill Cornell Medicine
New York

Sandeep K. Narang, MD, JD
Fulbright-Nehru Scholar 2014–2015
Division Head, Child Abuse Pediatrics
Ann & Robert H. Lurie Children's Hospital of Chicago
Associate Professor of Pediatrics
Northwestern Feinberg School of Medicine
Chicago, Illinois

Alice W. Newton, MD, FAAP
Medical Director, Child Protection Program
Massachusetts General Hospital for Children
Boston, Massachusetts

Gabriel Otterman, MD, MPH
Child Protection Team
Uppsala University Children's Hospital
Uppsala, Sweden

Vincent J. Palusci, MD, MS, FAAP
Professor of Pediatrics
NYU School of Medicine
New York

Robert M. Reece, MD, FAAP

Clinical Professor of Pediatrics, Tufts University School of Medicine (Retired)

Director, Child Protection Program

The Floating Hospital for Children

Tufts Medical Center

Boston, Massachusetts

Desmond K. Runyan, MD, DrPH, FACPM

National Program Director

Robert Wood Johnson Foundation Clinical Scholars

Jack and Viki Thompson Professor of Pediatrics

Executive Director Kempe Center for the Prevention and Treatment of Child Abuse and Neglect

The University of Colorado

Denver, Colorado

Lynn K. Sheets, MD, FAAP

Medical Director, Child Advocacy and Protection Services

Children's Hospital of Wisconsin

Professor, Medical College of Wisconsin

Section Chief, Child Advocacy and Protection

Milwaukee, Wisconsin

Suzanne P. Starling, MD, FAAP

Associate Director and Medical Director

Chadwick Center for Children and Families

Rady Children's Hospital San Diego

Clinical Professor of Pediatrics

University of California San Diego

San Diego, California

# References

## Chapter One

Caffey, J. I. 1946. "Multiple Fractures in the Long Bones of Infants Suffering from Chronic Subdural Hematoma." *American Journal of Roentgenology* 56: 163–173.

Feldman, Kenneth W., Robert T. Schaller, Jane A. Feldman, and Mollie McMillon. 1978. "Tap Water Scald Burns in Children." *Pediatrics* 62: 1–7.

Heins, Marilyn. 1984. "The 'Battered Child' Revisited." *Journal of the American Medical Association* 251: 3295–3300.

Kempe, C. Henry. 1978. "Sexual Abuse, Another Hidden Pediatric Problem: The 1977 C. Anderson Aldrich Lecture." *Pediatrics* 63: 382–389.

Kempe, C. Henry, Frederic N. Silverman, Brandt F. Steele, William Droegemueller, and Henry K. Silver. 1962. "The Battered-Child Syndrome." *Journal of the American Medical Association* 181: 17–24.

Labbe, Jean. 2005. "Ambroise Tardieu: The Man and His Work on Child Maltreatment a Century before Kempe." *Child Abuse & Neglect* 20: 311–324.

Lynch, Margaret A. 1985. "Child Abuse before Kempe: An Historical Literature Review." *Child Abuse & Neglect* 9: 7–15.

*Newsweek*. 1962, April 16. "When They're Angry." p. 74.

Ricci, Lawrence R., Cindy W. Christian, Robert M. Reece, Howard Dubowitz, and Steven Ludwig. 2002. "Report of the 1997 Child Abuse Physician Leadership Conference." *Child Maltreatment* 7: 166–169.

Roche, Albert J., Gilles Fortin, Jean Labbe, Jocelyn Brown, and David Chadwick. 2005. "The Work of Ambroise Tardieu: The First Definitive Description of Child Abuse." *Child Abuse & Neglect* 29: 235–334.

Silverman, Frederic N. 1953. "The Roentgen Manifestations of Unrecognized Skeletal Trauma in Infants." *American Journal of Roentgenology* 69: 413–427.

Silverman, Frederic N. 1994. "Letter to the Editor." *Pediatric Radiology* 24: 541–542.

Tardieu, Ambroise. 1857. "Etude medico-legale sur les attentants aux moeurs." Paris: Librairie JB Bailliere et Fils.

Tardieu, Ambroise. 1860. "Etude medico-legale sur les services at mauvais traitments exerces sur des enfants." *Annals d'Hygiene Publique et de Medecine Legale* 13: 361–398.

Tardieu, Ambroise. 1868. "Etude medico-legale sur l'infantcide." Paris: Librairie JB Bailoloiere et Fils.

## Chapter Two

Anderst, James, Nancy Kellogg, and Inkyung Jung. 2009. "Is the Diagnosis of Physical Abuse Changed When Child Protective Services Consults a Child Abuse Pediatrics Subspecialty Group as a Second Opinion?" *Child Abuse & Neglect* 33: 481–489.

Croskerry, Pat. 2002. "Achieving Quality in Clinical Decision Making: Cognitive Strategies and Detection of Bias." *Academic Emergency Medicine* 9: 11841204.

Croskerry, Pat. 2003. "The Importance of Cognitive Errors in Diagnosis and Strategies to Minimize Them." *Academic Medicine* 78: 775–780.

Dawson, Neal V., and Hal R. Arkes. 1987. "Systematic Errors in Medical Decision Making." *Journal of General Internal Medicine* 2: 183–187.

Flaherty, Emalee G., and Amanda K. Fingarson. 2012. "Child Physical Abuse: The Need for an Objective Assessment." *Pediatric Annals* 41: 411–415.

Flaherty, Emalee G., and Robert Sege. 2005. "Barriers to Physician Identification and Reporting of Child Abuse." *Pediatric Annals* 34: 349–356.

Jenny, Carole, Kent P. Hymel, Alene Ritzen, Steven E. Reinert, and Thomas C. Hay. 1999. "Analysis of Missed Cases of Abusive Head Trauma." *Journal of the American Medical Association* 281: 621–626.

Laskey, Antoinette L. 2014. "Cognitive Errors: Thinking Clearly When It Could Be Child Maltreatment." *Pediatric Clinics of North America* 61: 997–1005.

McGuire, Lindsay, Kimberly D. Martin, and John M. Leventhal. 2011. "Child Abuse Consultations Initiated by Child Protective Services: The Role of Expert Opinions." *Academic Pediatrics* 11: 467–473.

Sheets, Lynn K., Matthew E. Leach, Ian J. Koszewski, Ashley M. Lessmeier, Melodee Nugent, and Pippa Simpson. 2013. "Sentinel Injuries in Infants Evaluated for Child Physical Abuse." *Pediatrics* 131: 701–707.

Skellern, Catherine. 2015. "Minimizing Bias in the Forensic Evaluation of Suspicious Paediatric Injury." *Journal of Forensic and Legal Medicine* 34: 11–16.

## Chapter Three

Asher, Richard. 1951, February 10. "Munchausen's Syndrome." *The Lancet* 1(6650): 339–341.

Brown, Ana N., Gioia R. Gonzales, Rebecca T. Wiester, Maureen C. Kelley, and Kenneth W. Feldman. 2013. "Caretaker Blogs in Caregiver Fabricated

Illness in a Child: A Window on the Caretaker's Thinking." *Child Abuse & Neglect* 38: 488–497.

Bryk, Mary, and Patricia T. Siegel. 1997. "My Mother Caused My Illness: The Story of a Survivor of Munchausen by Proxy Syndrome." *Pediatrics* 100: 1–7.

Feldman, Kenneth W., David M. Christopher, and Kent B. Opheim. 1989. "Munchausen Syndrome/Bulimia by Proxy: Ipecac as a Toxin in Child Abuse." *Child Abuse & Neglect* 1089: 257–261.

Fleisher, David, and Marvin E. Ament. 1977. "Diarrhea, Red Diapers, and Child Abuse." *Clinical Pediatrics* 17: 820–824.

Hall, David E., Laura Eubanks, Swarnalatha Meyuyazhagan, Richard D. Kenney, and Sherry Cochran Johnson. 2000. "Evaluation of Covert Video Surveillance in the Diagnosis of Munchausen Syndrome by Proxy: Lessons from 42 Cases." *Pediatrics* 105: 1305–1312.

Meadow, Roy. 1977, August 13. "Munchausen Syndrome by Proxy: The Hinterland of Child Abuse." *The Lancet* 2(8033): 343–345.

Meadow, Roy. 1990. "Suffocation, Recurrent Apnea, and Sudden Infant Death." *Journal of Pediatrics* 117: 351–357.

Rosenberg, Donna A. 1987. "Web of Deceit: A Literature Review of Munchausen Syndrome by Proxy." *Child Abuse & Neglect* 11: 547–563.

Schreier, H. A. 1992. "The Perversion of Mothering: Munchausen Syndrome by Proxy." *Bulletin of Menninger Clinic* 56: 421–437.

Schreier, Herbert, and Lawrence R. Ricci. 2002. "Follow-Up of a Case of Munchausen by Proxy Syndrome." *Journal of the American Academy of Child and Adolescent Psychiatry* 41: 1395–1396.

Sugar, Jonathan A., Myron Belfer, Esther Israel, and David B. Herzog. 1991. "A 3-Year-Old Boy's Chronic Diarrhea and Unexplained Death." *Journal of the American Academy of Child and Adolescent Psychiatry* 30: 1015–1020.

## Chapter Four

Child Welfare Information Gateway. 2013. "Chronic Child Neglect." Washington, DC: U.S. Department of Health and Human Services, Children's Bureau.

Child Welfare Information Gateway. 2016. "Definitions of Child Abuse and Neglect." Washington, DC: U.S. Department of Health and Human Services, Children's Bureau. https://www.childwelfare.gov/topics/systemwide/laws-policies/statutes/define/.

Dubowitz, Howard. 2007. "Understanding and Addressing the 'Neglect of Neglect': Digging into the Molehill." *Child Abuse & Neglect* 31: 603–603.

Dubowitz, Howard, Angelo Giardino, and Edward Gustavson. 2000. "Child Neglect: Guidance for Pediatricians." *Pediatrics in Review* 21: 111–116.

Fong, Jiu-fai, and Cindy W. Christian. 2012. "Child Neglect: A Review for the Primary Care Pediatrician." *Pediatric Annals* 41: 1–5.

Green, Wayne H., Magda Campbell, and Raphael David. 1984. "Psychosocial Dwarfism: A Critical Review of the Evidence." *Journal of the American Academy of Child Psychiatry* 23: 39–48.

Sedlak, A. J., J. Mettenburg, M. Basena, I. Petta, K. McPherson, A. Greene, and S. Li. 2010. *Fourth National Incidence Study of Child Abuse and Neglect (NIS–4): Report to Congress.* Washington, DC: U.S. Department of Health and Human Services, Administration for Children and Families.

U.S. Department of Health and Human Services, Administration for Children and Families, Administration on Children, Youth and Families, Children's Bureau. 2016. *Child Maltreatment 2014.* http://www.acf.hhs.gov/programs/cb/research-data-technology/statistics-research/child-maltreatment.

Wolock, Isabel, and Bernard Horowitz. 1984. "Child Maltreatment as a Social Problem: The Neglect of Neglect." *American Journal of Orthopsychiatry* 54: 530–543.

## Chapter Five

Barr, Ronald G., Frederick P. Rivera, Marilyn Barr, Peter Cummings, James Taylor, Liliana J. Lengua, and Emily Meredith-Benitz. 2009. "Effectiveness of Educational Materials Designed to Change Knowledge and Behaviors Regarding Crying and Shaken-Baby Syndrome in Mothers of Newborns: A Randomized, Controlled Trial." *Pediatrics* 123: 972–980.

Commission to Eliminate Child Abuse and Neglect Fatalities. 2016. "Within Our Reach: A National Strategy to Eliminated Child Abuse and Neglect Fatalities." Washington, DC: Government Printing Office.

Dias, Mark S., Carroll M. Rottmund, Kelly M. Cappos, Marie E. Reed, Ming Wang, Christina Stetter, Michele L. Shaffer, Christopher S. Hollenbeak, Ian M. Paul, Cindy W. Christian, Rachel P. Berger, and Joanne Klevens. 2017. "Association of a Postnatal Parent Education Program for Abusive Head Trauma with Subsequent Pediatric Abusive Head Trauma Hospitalization Rates." *JAMA Pediatrics* 171: 223–229.

Dias, Mark S., Kim Smith, Kathy deGuehery, Paula Mazur, Veetai Li, and Michele L. Shaffer. 2005. "Preventing Abusive Head Trauma among Infants and Young Children: A Hospital-Based Parent Education Program." *Pediatrics* 115: e479-e477.

Donelan-McCall, Nancy, John Eckenrode, and David L. Olds. 2009. "Home Visiting for the Prevention of Child Maltreatment: Lessons Learned During the Past 20 Years." *Pediatric Clinics North America* 56: 389–403.

Every Child Matters Education Fund. 2010. "We Can Do Better: Child Abuse and Neglect Deaths in America." Washington, DC.

Farrell, Caitlin A., Eric W. Fleegler, Michael C. Monuteaux, Celeste R. Wilson, Cindy W. Christian, and Lois K. Lee. 2017. "Community Poverty and Child Abuse Fatalities in the United States." *Pediatrics* 139: e20161616.

Klevens, Joanne, Feijun Luo, Likang Xu, Cora Peterson, Natasha E. Latzman. 2016. "Paid Family Leave's Effect on Hospital Admissions for Pediatric Abusive Head Trauma." *Injury Prevention* 22: 442–445.

Krugman, Richard D. 1988. "Fatal Child Abuse: Analysis of 24 Cases." *Pediatrician* 12: 68–72.

Leventhal, John M. 2017. "Prevention of Pediatric Abusive Head Trauma: Time to Rethink Interventions and Reframe Messages." *JAMA Pediatrics* 171: 218–220.

Schnitzer, Patricia G., and Bernard G. Ewigman. 2005. "Child Deaths Resulting from Inflicted Injuries: Household Risk Factors and Perpetrator Characteristics." *Pediatrics* 116: 687–693.

Showers, Jacy. 1992. "Don't Shake the Baby: The Effectiveness of a Prevention Program." *Child Abuse & Neglect* 16: 11–18.

## Chapter Six

Commission to Eliminate Child Abuse and Neglect Fatalities. 2016. "Within Our Reach: A National Strategy to Eliminate Child Abuse and Neglect Fatalities." Washington, DC: Government Printing Office.

Gelles, Richard. 1996. *The Book of David: How Preserving Families Can Cost Children's Lives.* New York: Basic Books.

Jones, David P. H. 1987. "The Untreatable Family." *Child Abuse & Neglect* 11: 409–420.

Kim, Hyunil, Christopher Wilderman, Melissa Jonson-Reid, and Brett Drake. 2017. "Lifetime Prevalence of Investigating Child Maltreatment among US Children." *American Journal of Public Health* 107: 274–280.

Munro, Eileen. 1999. "Common Errors of Reasoning in Child Protective Work." *Child Abuse & Neglect* 23: 745–758.

U.S. Advisory Board on Child Abuse and Neglect. 1990. "Child Abuse and Neglect: Critical First Steps in Response to a National Emergency." Washington, DC: Government Printing Office.

## Chapter Eight

Block, Robert W. 1999 "Child Abuse—Controversies and Imposters." *Current Problems in Pediatrics* 29: 253–272.

Chadwick, David L. 1990. "Preparation for Court Testimony in Child Abuse Cases." *Pediatric Clinics of North America* 37: 955–970.

Myers, John E. B. 1992. *Legal Issues in Child Abuse and Neglect.* Newbury Park, CA: Sage Publications.

Paul, Stephan R., and Sandeep K. Narang. 2017. "Expert Witness Participation in Civil and Criminal Proceedings: Committee on Medical Liability and Risk Management." *Pediatrics* 139: e20163862.

St. Onge, Anita M., and Megan L. Elam. 2000. "Legal Intervention for the Physically Abused Child." In *Treatment of Child Abuse*, edited by Robert M. Reece, 107–116. Baltimore, MD: The Johns Hopkins University Press.

Stern, Paul. 1997. *Preparing and Presenting Expert Testimony in Child Abuse Litigation: A Guide for Expert Witnesses and Attorneys*. Thousand Oaks, CA: Sage Publications.

## Chapter Nine

McCann, Lisa, and Lori Anne Pearlman. 1990. "Vicarious Traumatization: A Framework for Understanding the Psychological Effect of Working with Victims." *Journal of Traumatic Stress* 3: 131–149.

Schetky, Diane, and Lesley Devoe. 1992. "Counter-Transference Issues in Forensic Child Psychiatry." In *Clinical Handbook of Child Psychiatry and the Law*, edited by Schetky and Benedek, 230–249. Baltimore, MD: Williams and Wilkins.

Simon, David. 1991. *Homicide: A Year on the Killing Streets*. New York: Henry Holt and Company.

# Index

Abusive head trauma, 19, 65–66, 93; annual incidence, 65; conference, 76; fatal, 30, 63; intent, 50; missed, 19, 86; screening tool, 108

Accidental injuries, 87, 114, 127

Acute Life Threatening Event (ALTE), 33

American Board of Pediatrics, 1, 5, 17

Anchoring, 20

Anderst, James, 22

Autopsy, 24, 30, 34, 44, 69, 71, 74, 115, 117, 118

Barron, Christine, 12–13, 40–41, 51, 66, 106–7, 125–27, 153

Battered child syndrome, 1–2, 4, 13

Berger, Rachel, 81–82, 124–25, 162

Bias, 20–22; anchoring, 20; availability, 20; confirmation, 20; counter transference, 123; feedback, 21; outcome, 20; premature closure, 22; visceral, 21

Block, Robert, 5–6, 153

The Book of David: How Preserving Families Can Cost Children's Lives, 80

Boos, Stephen, 112, 129–30, 143, 153

Brief Resolved Unexplained Events (BRUE), 33

Brown, Jocelyn, 139, 154

Brownell, Amanda, 11, 38–39, 107, 127–28, 154

Bryk, Mary, and chronic abuse, 37

Burns, 6–7, 13, 28, 53, 79

Caffey, John, 3–5

Child abuse diagnosis, court, 108

Child abuse diagnosis, missed, 19, 21–22

Child abuse diagnosis, mistakes, 19, 22

Child abuse diagnosis, research, 138

Child abuse fatal, 63–65, 81, 113, 119; causes, 63–64; incidence, 63–64; missed, 81; perpetrators, 78, 119; in 2014, 81

Child abuse fractures, 16, 25, 79; accidental, 138; brittle bone disease, 24; Caffey, 3; CPS MD Collaboration, 81; follow-up x-rays, 91; Kempe, Henry, 13

Child abuse investigation, 80

Child Abuse & Neglect: The International Journal, 2

Child abuse pediatricians, 2–3, 5, 8, 10, 14, 22; accuracy of diagnosis, 22–23; board certified, 22; mistakes, 21

Child abuse pediatrics, 1, 4–5, 17, 58, 143

Child abuse photo-documentation, 14–15

Child abuse research, 141, 144

Child Abuse Research, Education and Service Institute (CARES), 8

Child Protective Services (CPS), 5, 8, 22–25, 64, 85, 105, 152; reports, 144

Child welfare system, 21, 64, 83–85; family preservation, 80; rate of investigation, 80

Christian, Cindy, 5, 50, 145, 154

Commission to Eliminate Child Abuse and Neglect Fatalities, 64, 81

Counter transference, 123

Court, 104–5, 108; civil, 105; criminal, 104–5; expert testimony, 106, 111, 164; expert witness, 106–7, 163; material witness, 106; TV, 115, 116

CT scan, 73, 78, 121

Dubowitz, Howard, 5, 8–9, 47, 49, 84–85, 154

Failure to thrive, 13, 42, 43, 48–50, 51, 53, 55–56, 57, 58, 59, 60, 61, 130; definition, 50; intentional starvation, 59; nutritional, 49–50, 56, 60; psychosocial dwarfism, 57

Family Assessment Response (FAR), 139

Family risk factors, 14

Feldman, Kenneth, 6–7, 24–25, 38, 41–42, 84, 154

Finkel, Martin, 7–8, 129, 155

Flaherty, Emilee, 22, 37–38, 110, 155

*Forensic Study on Infanticide,* 2

*Forensic Study on Offenses against Morals,* 2

Fractures, 3, 14, 19, 20, 25; healing fractures, 13, 27, 28

Gelles, Richard, 80

Greeley, Christopher S., 146, 155

Helfer Society, 1, 9, 17, 143, 165

Hymel, Kent P., 10–11, 23–24, 108–10

International Society for the Prevention of Child Abuse and Neglect (ISPCAN), 2

International Society for the Prevention of Child Abuse and Neglect, Screening Tool (ICAST), 141

Jackson, Allison, 26–27, 39–40, 53–54, 83, 128–29, 155

Jenny, Carole, 10, 12, 19, 52–53, 82–83, 127, 155

Jones, David, 79

Kempe, Henry, 2, 4–5, 13, 17, 84, 143, 159; quoted in *Newsweek,* 4

Kerns, David, xiii

Krugman, Richard, 26, 51–52, 63, 67, 83–84, 156

Labbe, Jean, 1–2

Leventhal, John, 22, 65, 144, 156

Levin, Alex, 9–10, 25, 68, 108, 156

Ludwig, Stephen, 5, 9, 159

Maguire, Sabine, 137, 156

McCann, John, 25–26, 123, 157

Meadow, Roy, 35–36

Medical Child Abuse (MCA), 36, 38, 39, 41–42, 83, 131

Mian, Marcellina, 85, 130–31

Miller, Aaron, 142, 157

Mistakes, in child abuse, 17, 19–20, 23, 79, 81, 91; overdiagnosis, 19; underdiagnosis, 19

Multidisciplinary Team, 22, 66, 83, 140

Munchausen Syndrome by Proxy (Medical Child Abuse), 34–37, 45, 58, 161

"My Mother Caused My Illness: The Story of a Survivor of Munchausen by Proxy Syndrome," 37

Narang, Sandeep, 111–12, 157
National Center on Shaken Baby
    Syndrome, 65
National Child Abuse and Neglect
    Data Set (NCANDS), 47
National Incidence Study (NIS), 4
Neglect, 46, 141; definitions, 47;
    effects, 48; fatalities, 63–64, 81;
    incidence, 48; intent, 49–50
Nerwberger, Eli, 9
*Newsweek*, and Kempe, Henry, 4
Newton, Alice, 131, 157

Osteogenesis Imperfecta, 13, 25
Otterman, Gabriel, 140, 157

Palusci, Vincent, 157
*Pediatric Radiology*, 4
Period of Purple Crying Prevention
    Program, 65, 70, 75, 98, 123
Physical child abuse, 13, 22, 50
Poisoning: Ex-Lax, 43; ipecac, 40–41,
    42, 43
Prevention of child abuse, 137, 141,
    143–44, 147

Ray Helfer Society, 1, 9, 143, 165
Reece, Robert, 5, 158
Risk factors, 50, 63, 65

Rosenberg, Donna, 35–36, 161
Runyan, Desmond, 68–69, 85, 140,
    158

Sentinel injury, 28, 86, 160
Sexual abuse, 2, 4, 25, 49, 112, 123,
    127, 139, 141–42, 159
"Sexual Abuse, Another Hidden
    Pediatric Problem," 4
Sgroi, Suzanne, 7
Shaken baby syndrome, 65, 69, 76,
    93, 98, 123
Sheets, Lynn, 27–28, 110–11, 158
Silverman, Frederic, 3–5
Starling, Suzanne, 113–14, 158

Tardieu, Ambroise, 1–5, 17

United Nations Children's Fund
    (UNICEF), 142–43
United States Air Force (USAF)
    medical corps, 10
"The Untreatable Family," 79
U.S. Advisory Board on Child Abuse
    and Neglect, 83

Vicarious trauma, 123–24

"Web of Deceit" syndrome, 35–36

## About the Author

**Lawrence R. Ricci, MD**, is board-certified in pediatrics and child abuse pediatrics. He is a clinical professor of pediatrics at the Tufts University School of Medicine. Ricci specializes in the evaluation and treatment of abused children as medical director of the Spurwink Child Abuse Program in Maine. He is also on the consulting staff at Barbara Bush Children's Hospital, where, in addition to evaluating inpatients for abuse, he trains medical students and pediatric residents in detecting child abuse. Ricci is a former chair of the section on Child Abuse of the American Academy of Pediatrics. He is a former president of the Ray Helfer Society, an honorary society of several hundred physicians from around the world specializing in the care of abused children. Ricci has developed numerous child abuse workshops that have been presented to social workers, mental health professionals, legal professionals, and medical professionals across the nation. He has been the recipient of multiple awards including the American Academy of Pediatrics Section on Child Abuse award for Outstanding Service to Abused Children, and the Ray Helfer Society award for Outstanding Service to the Field of Child Abuse Pediatrics.